THE SATTVIC DIET

BALANCING BODY, MIND, AND SPIRIT

CONTENTS

INTRODUCTION

Welcome to "The Sattvic Diet: Balancing Body, Mind, and Spirit." In the modern world, where hectic lifestyles and stress often take center stage, finding a way to achieve balance and well-being can seem elusive. However, the Sattvic diet offers a profound path to reconnecting with our innate harmony and experiencing holistic wellness.

Derived from ancient wisdom and rooted in the principles of Ayurveda and yoga, the Sattvic diet presents a holistic approach to nourishing the body, mind, and spirit. It goes beyond mere sustenance and embraces the idea that the food we consume directly influences our overall well-being, affecting not only our physical health but also our mental and spiritual states.

In this comprehensive guide, we embark on a transformative journey to understand and embrace the principles and philosophy of the Sattvic diet. We delve into its origins, exploring the rich heritage of the ancient Indus Valley civilization and the sacred texts that have passed down this wisdom through the ages. We uncover the guiding principles that govern the Sattvic diet, discovering how the interplay of the three Gunas—Sattva, Rajas, and Tamas—affects our being.

With a focus on achieving balance and bliss, we explore the profound benefits that the Sattvic diet offers. From supporting physical health and vitality to nurturing mental clarity and emotional balance, this dietary approach encompasses a wide spectrum of well-being. Additionally, we delve into the spiritual dimensions of the Sattvic diet, understanding how it can serve as a catalyst for spiritual growth and awakening.

Throughout this book, we not only provide you with practical insights into incorporating Sattvic principles into your dietary choices but also guide you in integrating this lifestyle into your everyday routine. From planning balanced Sattvic meals and exploring nourishing recipes to incorporating Sattvic herbs and spices and engaging in mindfulness practices, we equip you with the tools and knowledge to embark on a journey of holistic transformation.

By embracing the Sattvic diet, you have the opportunity to harmonize your body, mind, and spirit, fostering a state of well-being that radiates from within. Prepare to embark on this enlightening journey as we delve into the depths of the Sattvic diet, unveiling the path to balance, vitality, and blissful living.

1. UNDERSTANDING THE SATTVIC DIET: PRINCIPLES AND PHILOSOPHY

The term "Sattvic" comes from the ancient Indian philosophy of Ayurveda and yoga. In Sanskrit, "Sattva" refers to a state of purity, balance, and harmony. It represents qualities such as clarity, calmness, contentment, and spiritual awareness. The Sattvic state is associated with a sense of inner peace and tranquility.

In the context of the Sattvic diet, "Sattvic" refers to the foods and lifestyle practices that promote Sattva or the Sattvic state of being. The Sattvic diet is a way of eating that aims to cultivate these qualities of purity, balance, and harmony within the body, mind, and spirit. It emphasizes consuming foods that are considered pure, fresh, light, and naturally sourced from the earth. The Sattvic diet focuses on nourishing the body while promoting mental clarity, emotional stability, and spiritual growth.

The Sattvic lifestyle extends beyond food choices and includes practices such as meditation, yoga, self-reflection, and conscious living. It encourages individuals to cultivate a state of awareness, mindfulness, and compassion in their daily lives. The Sattvic approach is considered beneficial for promoting overall well-being, supporting a balanced state of mind, and enhancing spiritual growth.

By embracing the Sattvic philosophy, individuals strive to align themselves with the principles of purity, balance, and harmony, not just in their dietary choices but also in their thoughts, actions, and interactions with others and the world around them. The goal is to create a harmonious integration of body, mind, and spirit, leading to a state of holistic wellness and inner peace.

The Sattvic diet is a dietary approach rooted in ancient Indian philosophy and Ayurveda, a holistic system of medicine and well-being. It is based on the principles of Sattva, one of the three Gunas (qualities) described in Hindu philosophy. Sattva represents purity, harmony, and balance. The Sattvic diet aims to cultivate these qualities in both body and mind, promoting overall health, clarity, and spiritual growth.

1.1 PRINCIPLES OF THE SATTVIC DIET:

Pure and Fresh Foods: The Sattvic diet emphasizes the consumption of pure, fresh, and unprocessed foods. This includes fruits, vegetables, whole grains, nuts, seeds, legumes, dairy products (in moderation), and natural sweeteners. These foods are considered to be rich in prana, the vital life force, and are believed to nourish the body and mind.

Sattvic Food Qualities: Sattvic foods are characterized by their lightness, clarity, and high nutritional value. They are believed to promote mental clarity and spiritual awareness. Sattvic foods are ideally grown organically, without the use of pesticides or chemical fertilizers, and are prepared with love and mindfulness.

Satvic Mindset: The Sattvic diet goes beyond food choices; it encompasses a holistic lifestyle approach. Practitioners of the Sattvic diet are encouraged to cultivate a Sattvic mindset by practicing mindfulness, compassion, and self-awareness. This involves avoiding negative influences, such as violent or disturbing media, and fostering positive thoughts and behaviors.

Ahimsa (Non-violence): Ahimsa is a core principle of the Sattvic diet. It promotes the idea of non-violence and compassion towards all living beings. As such, a Sattvic diet avoids foods derived from the harm or killing of animals, such as meat, fish, and eggs. Instead, it encourages plant-based alternatives for protein and other essential nutrients.

Moderation and Balance: The Sattvic diet emphasizes the importance of moderation and balance in eating habits. Overeating and excessive indulgence are discouraged, as they are believed to disrupt the equilibrium of the body and mind. Eating mindfully, chewing food thoroughly, and listening to the body's hunger and satiety signals are essential practices in the Sattvic diet.

1.2 BENEFITS OF THE SATTVIC DIET:

Improved Digestion: The emphasis on fresh, whole foods and mindful eating practices in the Sattvic diet can promote healthy digestion. This can help alleviate digestive issues, improve nutrient absorption, and support overall gut health.

Enhanced Mental Clarity: Sattvic foods are considered to have a calming effect on the mind, promoting mental clarity and focus. By avoiding processed and heavy foods, which can lead to lethargy and brain fog, practitioners of the Sattvic diet aim to maintain a state of alertness and clarity.

Increased Vitality: Sattvic foods are typically rich in essential nutrients, vitamins, and minerals, which provide the body with sustained energy and vitality. The diet's emphasis on fresh fruits and vegetables, whole grains, and plant-based proteins helps nourish the body and support overall well-being.

Emotional Balance: The Sattvic diet promotes emotional balance and stability. It encourages the consumption of foods that are believed to have a positive impact on the mind, reducing negative emotions and promoting feelings of peace, compassion, and contentment.

Spiritual Growth: The Sattvic diet is closely linked to spiritual practices and aims to support spiritual growth and self-realization. By consuming pure and light foods, practitioners believe they can elevate their consciousness and develop a deeper connection to their inner self and the universe.

It's important to note that the Sattvic diet may not be suitable for everyone. Individual dietary needs, health conditions, and cultural backgrounds should be taken into consideration. It is always advisable to consult with a healthcare professional or a registered dietitian before making significant changes to your diet.

Quite simply, the Sattvic diet is a dietary approach deeply rooted in the principles of Ayurveda and Hindu philosophy. It promotes the consumption of pure, fresh, and unprocessed foods, mindfulness in eating habits, and a compassionate mindset. By adhering to the Sattvic diet, individuals aim to cultivate physical and mental well-being, clarity, and spiritual growth.

1.3 ORIGINS AND PHILOSOPHY OF THE SATTVIC DIET

The Sattvic diet finds its origins in ancient Indian philosophy and Ayurveda, a traditional system of medicine that emphasizes the balance between body, mind, and spirit. The term "Sattvic" comes from the Sanskrit word "Sattva," which means purity, harmony, and balance. It is one of the three Gunas or qualities described in Hindu philosophy, the other two being Rajas (activity/passion) and Tamas (inertia/darkness). The Sattvic diet aims to cultivate the Sattva quality and promote overall well-being on physical, mental, and spiritual levels.

The philosophy behind the Sattvic diet is deeply rooted in the idea of holistic health, where the food we consume directly affects our physical and mental states. According to Ayurveda, our bodies are composed of five elements: earth, water, fire, air, and space. These elements combine to form three doshas or energies: Vata (air and space), Pitta (fire and water), and Kapha (earth and water). The Sattvic diet is considered ideal for balancing these doshas and maintaining overall equilibrium in the body.

The Sattvic diet emphasizes the consumption of pure, fresh, and unprocessed foods that are considered to be rich in prana, the vital life force. This includes fruits, vegetables, whole grains, nuts, seeds, legumes, dairy products (in moderation), and natural sweeteners. Sattvic foods are believed to be light and easy to digest, providing nourishment to the body without causing heaviness or lethargy.

One of the fundamental principles of the Sattvic diet is Ahimsa, which means non-violence or compassion towards all living beings. This principle extends to the food choices made by practitioners of the Sattvic diet. They avoid foods derived from the harm or killing of animals, such as meat, fish, and eggs, and instead opt for plant-based alternatives. By doing so, they aim to cultivate a sense of compassion, minimize harm to other beings, and promote harmony with nature.

The Sattvic diet also promotes moderation and balance in eating habits. Overeating and excessive indulgence are discouraged as they are believed to disrupt the equilibrium of the body and mind. Practitioners are encouraged to eat mindfully, chewing their food thoroughly, and listening to their body's hunger and satiety signals.

Beyond food choices, the Sattvic diet encourages a Sattvic mindset and lifestyle. Practitioners are advised to practice mindfulness, meditation, and self-awareness. They are encouraged to cultivate positive thoughts, engage in activities that promote mental and emotional well-being, and avoid negative influences such as violent or disturbing media. By adopting these practices, individuals aim to develop a greater sense of inner peace, clarity, and spiritual growth.

The benefits of following a Sattvic diet are believed to extend to both physical and mental well-being. By consuming fresh and unprocessed foods, practitioners can obtain a wide range of essential nutrients, vitamins, and minerals necessary for optimal health. The diet's emphasis on plant-based foods and avoidance of heavy or processed foods can help improve digestion, support healthy weight management, and enhance vitality.

Mentally, the Sattvic diet is thought to promote clarity, focus, and emotional balance. The consumption of light and pure foods is believed to have a calming effect on the mind, reducing negative emotions and promoting feelings of peace, compassion, and contentment. By adopting a Sattvic lifestyle, individuals can enhance their overall sense of well-being and spiritual growth.

It is important to note that the Sattvic diet is not a one-size-fits-all approach. Individual dietary needs, health conditions, and cultural backgrounds should be taken into consideration. It is always advisable to consult with a healthcare professional or a registered dietitian before making significant changes to your diet.

In conclusion, the Sattvic diet is rooted in ancient Indian philosophy and Ayurveda, emphasizing the principles of purity, harmony, and balance. It promotes the consumption of fresh, unprocessed, and plant-based foods, while discouraging the consumption of animal-derived products and heavy or processed foods. By following the Sattvic diet and embracing a Sattvic lifestyle, individuals aim to achieve physical, mental, and spiritual well-being.

1.4 THE THREE GUNAS: SATTVA, RAJAS, AND TAMAS

The Sattvic diet finds its origins in ancient Indian philosophy and Ayurveda, a traditional system of medicine that emphasizes the balance between body, mind, and spirit. The term "Sattvic" comes from the Sanskrit word "Sattva," which means purity, harmony, and balance. It is one of the three Gunas or qualities described in Hindu philosophy, the other two being Rajas (activity/passion) and Tamas (inertia/darkness). In ancient Indian philosophy, the concept of the three Gunas—Sattva, Rajas, and Tamas—provides a framework for understanding the nature of existence and the qualities that shape the world and individual experiences. These Gunas are believed to be the fundamental energies or forces that underlie all aspects of life, including human behavior, thoughts, emotions, and the entire universe. Understanding the characteristics and interplay of these Gunas can offer insights into the complexities of human nature and guide individuals towards balance and self-realization.

Sattva:

Sattva is the highest and purest Guna, representing qualities of purity, harmony, and balance. It is associated with light, clarity, knowledge, wisdom, and spiritual awareness. When Sattva is dominant, individuals experience inner peace, contentment, and a sense of well-being. Sattvic qualities include compassion, truthfulness, self-discipline, love, and serenity. The Sattvic state of mind is characterized by a clear perception of reality, positive thoughts, and an overall balanced and virtuous approach to life.

In terms of diet, Sattva is reflected in the Sattvic diet, which emphasizes the consumption of pure, fresh, and unprocessed foods. These foods are believed to nourish the body and mind, promote mental clarity, and support spiritual growth. The Sattvic diet includes fruits, vegetables, whole grains, nuts, seeds, legumes, dairy products (in moderation), and natural sweeteners.

Rajas:

Rajas is the Guna associated with activity, passion, and restlessness. It represents the driving force that fuels ambition, desires, and the pursuit of worldly goals. Rajas is characterized by action, movement, and stimulation. It can manifest as intense emotions, attachment, and a tendency towards materialism. When Rajas is dominant, individuals may experience excitement, ambition, and a need for achievement. However, excessive Rajas can lead to overactivity, stress, and a scattered mind.

Rajas is often associated with the modern lifestyle, where constant stimulation and a fast-paced environment prevail. In terms of diet, Rajas is reflected in foods that are stimulating and energizing, such as spicy or heavily seasoned dishes, caffeinated beverages, and foods high in sugar or additives. While Rajas can be necessary for motivation and productivity, it is important to cultivate a balanced approach and prevent it from overpowering the other Gunas.

Tamas:

Tamas is the Guna associated with darkness, inertia, and ignorance. It represents qualities of heaviness, dullness, and resistance to change. Tamas is characterized by laziness, lethargy, confusion, and a lack of clarity. When Tamas dominates, individuals may experience inertia, apathy, and a lack of motivation. Tamas can also manifest as negative emotions, ignorance, and destructive behaviors.

In terms of diet, Tamas is reflected in foods that are heavy, processed, and difficult to digest. These include deep-fried foods, processed meats, excessive amounts of refined sugars, and foods with low nutritional value. Consuming Tamasic foods is believed to dull the mind, hinder clarity, and contribute to feelings of sluggishness and lethargy.

The interplay of these three Gunas is dynamic and ever-changing. Each individual has a unique combination and varying degrees of these Gunas, which can influence their thoughts, emotions, behaviors, and overall state of being. The goal is not to eliminate any particular Guna but to cultivate awareness and strive for balance.

Practices such as yoga, meditation, self-reflection, and mindful living can help individuals become more aware of the Gunas within themselves and in the world around them. By cultivating Sattva, individuals can strive for clarity, wisdom, and spiritual growth. By managing Rajas, individuals can direct their energy towards productive and positive pursuits. And by reducing Tamas, individuals can overcome inertia and ignorance, and awaken to their true potential.

the concept of the three Gunas—Sattva, Rajas, and Tamas—provides a profound understanding of the nature of existence and the qualities that shape human experiences. By recognizing the interplay of these Gunas within ourselves and making conscious choices, we can strive for balance, self-realization, and a harmonious way of living.

1.5 BENEFITS OF EMBRACING A SATTVIC LIFESTYLE

Embracing a Sattvic lifestyle, which encompasses not only dietary choices but also overall mindset and practices, can have profound benefits for individuals seeking to achieve harmony and well-being. By aligning the body, mind, and spirit, and cultivating qualities of purity, balance, and compassion, practitioners can experience a range of positive effects. Let's explore the benefits of embracing a Sattvic lifestyle in more detail:

Physical Well-being:

One of the primary benefits of a Sattvic lifestyle is improved physical health. The emphasis on consuming fresh, unprocessed, and plant-based foods provides the body with a rich array of essential nutrients, vitamins, and minerals. These nutrients support overall vitality, boost the immune system, and enhance bodily functions. The Sattvic diet, with its focus on light and easily digestible foods, can also promote efficient digestion, prevent digestive disorders, and support healthy weight management.

Mental Clarity and Emotional Balance:

A Sattvic lifestyle is known to promote mental clarity, emotional balance, and inner peace. The consumption of pure and light foods is believed to have a positive impact on the mind, reducing negative emotions and promoting feelings of calmness and serenity. By avoiding heavy and processed foods, practitioners can minimize brain fog and enhance mental focus, clarity, and concentration. The practice of mindfulness and self-awareness, encouraged in a Sattvic lifestyle, can also help individuals manage stress, anxiety, and negative thought patterns.

Spiritual Growth and Self-Realization:

The Sattvic lifestyle places a strong emphasis on spirituality and self-realization. By cultivating qualities such as compassion, truthfulness, and love, practitioners can deepen their spiritual connection and sense of purpose. The consumption of Sattvic foods, believed to be filled with vital life force or prana, can support the purification and balance of energy centers within the body, known as chakras. This purification is said to enhance spiritual growth and facilitate a greater understanding of oneself and the interconnectedness of all beings.

Enhanced Energy and Vitality:

Following a Sattvic lifestyle can lead to increased energy levels and overall vitality. The consumption of fresh, natural foods provides the body with essential nutrients, while avoiding processed and heavy foods prevents energy drains and sluggishness. Sattvic practices, such as yoga, pranayama (breathing exercises), and meditation, can also rejuvenate the body and mind, promote optimal energy flow, and boost overall vitality.

Cultivation of Compassion and Harmony:

Central to the Sattvic lifestyle is the principle of Ahimsa, or non-violence and compassion towards all beings. By choosing a plant-based diet and avoiding foods derived from the harm or killing of animals, individuals cultivate a sense of empathy, compassion, and harmony with the natural world. This compassionate mindset extends beyond food choices and influences interactions with others, promoting harmonious relationships and a sense of interconnectedness.

Environmental Sustainability:

Embracing a Sattvic lifestyle aligns with principles of environmental sustainability. By consuming plant-based, locally sourced, and organic foods, practitioners reduce their ecological footprint and contribute to the well-being of the planet. The emphasis on mindful consumption and avoiding excessive waste fosters a greater awareness of environmental impact and encourages responsible choices.

Overall Well-being:

By embracing a Sattvic lifestyle, individuals can experience a holistic sense of well-being. The balance and harmony cultivated through Sattvic practices can positively impact physical health, mental clarity, emotional balance, and spiritual growth. By aligning the body, mind, and spirit and adopting a compassionate mindset, practitioners can lead fulfilling and purposeful lives.

It's important to note that the benefits of a Sattvic lifestyle may vary from person to person, and it is always advisable to seek personalized guidance from healthcare professionals or qualified practitioners of Ayurveda or holistic medicine.

Embracing a Sattvic lifestyle offers numerous benefits, encompassing physical health, mental clarity, emotional balance, spiritual growth, and environmental sustainability. By aligning the body, mind, and spirit and adopting practices that promote purity, balance, and compassion, individuals can experience a profound sense of well-being and harmony in their lives.

2. EXPLORING THE SATTVIC MINDSET: CULTIVATING INNER HARMONY

The Sattvic mindset is an integral aspect of the Sattvic lifestyle, focusing on cultivating inner harmony and balance. It involves adopting a specific approach to life and nurturing qualities that promote clarity, peace, and spiritual growth. By embracing the Sattvic mindset, individuals can attain a deeper understanding of themselves, their interactions with others, and their connection to the world around them. Let's delve into the key aspects of the Sattvic mindset and how they contribute to inner harmony:

Self-awareness:

At the core of the Sattvic mindset lies self-awareness—the ability to observe and understand one's thoughts, emotions, and behaviors without judgment. Self-awareness allows individuals to recognize their own patterns, beliefs, and conditioning, enabling them to make conscious choices that align with their true nature. Through practices such as meditation, reflection, and introspection, individuals can cultivate self-awareness and develop a deeper understanding of themselves.

Clarity of thought:

A Sattvic mindset promotes clarity of thought by encouraging individuals to examine their beliefs, opinions, and perceptions. It involves questioning assumptions and exploring alternative perspectives. By fostering clarity, individuals can make informed decisions, navigate challenges effectively, and maintain mental focus. Practices such as mindfulness meditation and contemplation aid in quieting the mind, reducing mental chatter, and attaining a state of clarity.

Cultivation of inner peace:

Inner peace is a central aspect of the Sattvic mindset. It involves finding tranquility amidst the ups and downs of life. By nurturing a sense of inner calm, individuals can navigate stress, anxiety, and uncertainty with greater resilience. Sattvic practices like yoga, breathwork (pranayama), and meditation help calm the nervous system, reduce stress hormones, and cultivate a state of peace within.

Compassion and empathy:

The Sattvic mindset emphasizes the cultivation of compassion and empathy towards oneself and others. Compassion involves extending kindness, understanding, and support to oneself and those around them. It fosters a sense of connection and unity with all beings. By practicing acts of kindness, gratitude, and selflessness, individuals develop a compassionate mindset that promotes harmonious relationships and a sense of collective well-being.

Detachment:

Detachment, in the Sattvic context, refers to the ability to let go of attachments to outcomes, possessions, and ego-driven desires. It involves embracing a mindset of non-attachment and surrendering to the flow of life. Detachment does not imply indifference or apathy, but rather a sense of freedom from clinging to transient aspects of life. By cultivating detachment, individuals can experience a greater sense of inner peace, contentment, and acceptance of the present moment.

Intentional living:

A Sattvic mindset encourages intentional living, where individuals align their actions and choices with their values and higher purpose. It involves making conscious decisions regarding lifestyle, relationships, and the use of time and resources. By living with intention, individuals create a life that is in harmony with their authentic selves and promotes personal growth and fulfillment.

Spiritual growth:

The Sattvic mindset is closely tied to spiritual growth and self-realization. It involves a deepening connection to the inner self and a recognition of the interconnectedness of all beings. By embracing spiritual practices such as meditation, contemplation, and self-inquiry, individuals can cultivate a profound sense of spiritual awareness, expand their consciousness, and align with their higher purpose.

By embracing the Sattvic mindset and incorporating these principles into daily life, individuals can cultivate inner harmony, clarity, and peace. It is important to remember that developing a Sattvic mindset is a journey that requires patience, self-compassion, and consistent practice. Over time, individuals can experience a transformation in their outlook, relationships, and overall well-being, leading to a more fulfilled and purposeful life.

Remember, the Sattvic mindset is a personal exploration, and each individual's journey will be unique. It is advisable to seek guidance from experienced practitioners, spiritual teachers, or mentors who can provide insights and support along the way.

Becoming Self Aware

Becoming self-aware is a transformative process that involves conscious introspection and reflection. Under the Sattvic teachings, self-awareness is considered a fundamental aspect of personal growth and spiritual development. Here are some steps to cultivate self-awareness and assess if you are truly self-aware within the Sattvic teachings:

Practice mindfulness: Mindfulness is the foundation of self-awareness. Cultivate the habit of being fully present in the present moment, observing your thoughts, emotions, and sensations without judgment. Regular mindfulness meditation helps develop the skill of introspection and enhances self-awareness.

Engage in self-reflection: Set aside dedicated time for self-reflection. This can involve journaling, contemplation, or engaging in activities that promote introspection, such as walking in nature or practicing silence. Reflect on your thoughts, beliefs, emotions, and behaviors, aiming to understand their origins and patterns.

Seek feedback from others: Reach out to trusted friends, family members, or mentors who can provide honest feedback about your behavior, strengths, and areas for improvement. Actively listen to their perspectives and be open to constructive criticism. This external feedback can shed light on aspects of yourself that you may not be fully aware of.

Practice self-inquiry: Ask yourself deeper questions to explore your beliefs, values, and motivations. Reflect on your desires, fears, and aspirations. Question the assumptions and biases that shape your worldview. Self-inquiry encourages introspection and uncovers hidden aspects of yourself.

Observe your reactions: Pay attention to how you respond to different situations, both pleasant and challenging. Observe your emotional reactions, thought patterns, and behavioral tendencies. Notice if there are recurring patterns or triggers that elicit certain reactions. This observation allows you to gain insights into your inner world and automatic responses.

Cultivate non-judgmental awareness: As you develop self-awareness, practice cultivating a non-judgmental attitude towards yourself. Avoid labeling your thoughts, emotions, or behaviors as "good" or "bad." Instead, aim to observe them with curiosity and compassion. This attitude creates a safe space for self-exploration and growth.

Practice self-acceptance: Embrace all aspects of yourself, including your strengths, weaknesses, and imperfections. Acceptance is an essential part of self-awareness and personal growth. Recognize that self-awareness is not about attaining perfection but rather about developing a deeper understanding and acceptance of who you are.

To assess if you are truly self-aware under the Sattvic teachings, consider the following indicators:

Are you able to observe your thoughts, emotions, and behaviors without immediate reactivity?

Do you have an understanding of your core values and beliefs?

Are you able to recognize and manage your own emotions effectively?

Do you notice patterns in your thoughts, emotions, and behaviors and take steps to address any negative or unhelpful patterns?

Are you open to feedback from others and willing to explore areas of improvement?

Do you have a sense of purpose and alignment with your higher values?

Remember that self-awareness is a lifelong practice, and it deepens over time with continued effort and self-reflection. Embracing the Sattvic teachings and incorporating mindfulness, self-inquiry, and compassion into your daily life can support your journey towards genuine self-awareness.

2.1 DEVELOPING MENTAL CLARITY AND EMOTIONAL BALANCE

In the fast-paced and complex world we live in, developing mental clarity and emotional balance is essential for our overall well-being. These qualities enable us to navigate challenges, make wise decisions, and cultivate inner peace. Within the context of the Sattvic teachings, mental clarity and emotional balance are seen as integral aspects of a balanced and harmonious life. Let's explore how we can develop and nurture these qualities:

Mindfulness Meditation:

Mindfulness meditation is a powerful practice for developing mental clarity and emotional balance. By training our attention to focus on the present moment without judgment, we cultivate awareness of our thoughts, emotions, and sensations. Regular mindfulness practice helps us observe the fluctuations of the mind and develop the ability to let go of distractions and mental chatter. This cultivates mental clarity and a sense of calmness.

Breath Awareness:

Conscious breath awareness is a simple yet effective technique for developing mental clarity and emotional balance. By bringing our attention to the breath, we anchor ourselves in the present moment and calm the mind. Deep, slow breathing activates the parasympathetic nervous system, promoting relaxation and reducing stress. This practice enhances mental clarity and supports emotional equilibrium.

Self-Reflection and Journaling:

Engaging in self-reflection and journaling allows us to explore our thoughts, emotions, and experiences in a deeper and more conscious way. By regularly reflecting on our inner world, we gain insight into our patterns, beliefs, and reactions. This process helps us identify areas where mental clarity may be lacking and enables us to bring conscious awareness to our emotional states. Writing down our thoughts and feelings can provide clarity, emotional release, and a greater understanding of ourselves.

Cultivating a Balanced Lifestyle:

A balanced lifestyle plays a crucial role in developing mental clarity and emotional balance. Adequate rest, sufficient sleep, regular exercise, and a nutritious diet all contribute to overall well-being. When we take care of our physical health, we provide a solid foundation for mental and emotional well-being. The Sattvic diet, consisting of fresh, plant-based foods, promotes physical vitality, clarity of mind, and emotional stability.

Emotional Regulation:

Developing emotional regulation skills is vital for achieving emotional balance. It involves recognizing and understanding our emotions, as well as learning how to respond to them in a healthy and constructive manner. Techniques such as deep breathing, mindfulness, and self-compassion can help us navigate challenging emotions with grace and clarity. Cultivating empathy and self-awareness also allows us to understand the underlying causes of our emotions and respond with greater compassion towards ourselves and others.

Clear Communication:

Clear and effective communication supports mental clarity and emotional balance in our relationships. When we express ourselves authentically and listen attentively to others, we reduce misunderstandings and conflicts. Honest and compassionate communication promotes understanding, harmony, and emotional well-being. Developing active listening skills and practicing non-violent communication techniques can enhance our ability to communicate clearly and empathetically.

Limiting Distractions:

In today's digital age, it's important to consciously limit distractions that can hinder mental clarity and emotional balance. Excessive use of technology, constant multitasking, and information overload can overwhelm the mind and lead to scattered thoughts and emotional turbulence. Setting boundaries with technology, carving out designated periods of uninterrupted time, and engaging in activities that promote focus and concentration (e.g., reading, practicing art, or spending time in nature) can support mental clarity and emotional equilibrium.

Cultivating Gratitude and Positive Mindset:

Practicing gratitude and cultivating a positive mindset contribute to mental clarity and emotional balance. Regularly acknowledging and appreciating the blessings, opportunities, and positive aspects of life helps shift our perspective and counteracts negativity. Gratitude practices, such as keeping a gratitude journal or expressing gratitude to others, promote a sense of contentment, joy, and mental clarity. Positive affirmations and intentional reframing of negative thoughts can also support a positive mindset and emotional balance.

By incorporating these practices into our daily lives, we can develop mental clarity and emotional balance. It's important to remember that these qualities require consistent effort, patience, and self-compassion. Embracing the Sattvic teachings, which emphasize purity, balance, and self-awareness, can further support our journey toward mental clarity and emotional well-being.

2.2 MEDITATION AND MINDFULNESS PRACTICES

Meditation and mindfulness practices have gained widespread popularity in recent years as effective tools for reducing stress, promoting well-being, and cultivating a deeper sense of self-awareness. Within the context of the Sattvic teachings, meditation and mindfulness are considered integral practices for attaining spiritual growth, mental clarity, and inner harmony. Let's explore the various forms of meditation and mindfulness practices and their benefits:

Mindfulness Meditation:

Mindfulness meditation is a form of meditation that involves bringing non-judgmental awareness to the present moment. It is about intentionally paying attention to our thoughts, emotions, bodily sensations, and the surrounding environment. By cultivating this open and non-reactive awareness, we develop a deeper understanding of ourselves and the world around us. Mindfulness meditation helps us break free from automatic patterns of thinking and reacting, leading to greater mental clarity, emotional balance, and a sense of inner peace.

Breath Awareness Meditation:

Breath awareness meditation is a foundational practice that involves focusing one's attention on the breath. By observing the natural rhythm of the breath without trying to control it, we anchor ourselves in the present moment and cultivate a state of relaxation and centeredness. This practice enhances concentration, reduces stress, and promotes a sense of clarity and calmness. Breath awareness meditation can be practiced in various ways, such as focusing on the sensation of the breath at the nostrils or the rising and falling of the abdomen.

Loving-Kindness Meditation:

Loving-kindness meditation, also known as Metta meditation, is a practice that involves cultivating feelings of love, compassion, and goodwill towards oneself and others. It typically starts with directing positive intentions and well-wishes towards oneself, then gradually extending those wishes to loved ones, neutral individuals, and even difficult or challenging individuals. This practice helps develop empathy, forgiveness, and a sense of interconnectedness. Loving-kindness meditation fosters emotional balance, reduces negativity, and promotes a deep sense of inner peace and connection.

Mantra Meditation:

Mantra meditation involves the repetition of a specific word, phrase, or sound (mantra) to focus and quiet the mind. The chosen mantra can be a sacred word, a meaningful affirmation, or a sound with no specific meaning. By repeating the mantra, either silently or aloud, we create a point of concentration that helps calm the mind and induce a meditative state. Mantra meditation cultivates mental clarity, deep relaxation, and can serve as a powerful tool for spiritual transformation.

Walking Meditation:

Walking meditation is a form of meditation that involves bringing mindfulness and awareness to the act of walking. It can be practiced indoors or outdoors, in a slow and deliberate manner.

The focus is on the sensations of walking—the movement of the feet, the contact with the ground, and the rhythmic flow of the body. Walking meditation promotes grounding, embodiment, and mindfulness in motion. It can be a refreshing practice that combines meditation, physical activity, and connection with nature.

Body Scan Meditation:

Body scan meditation involves systematically bringing attention to different parts of the body, noticing physical sensations, and cultivating a sense of relaxation and presence. Starting from the top of the head and moving downward, or vice versa, one directs attention to each part of the body, observing any tension, discomfort, or sensations without judgment. Body scan meditation helps develop body awareness, reduces stress, and promotes a sense of physical and mental well-being.

Visualization Meditation:

Visualization meditation involves creating mental images or scenarios to evoke specific feelings, qualities, or desired outcomes. Guided imagery or visualization practices can be used to cultivate positive emotions, enhance creativity, improve focus, or envision personal goals. Visualization meditation can be particularly helpful for enhancing mental clarity, developing a positive mindset, and manifesting intentions.

Open Awareness Meditation:

Open awareness meditation involves simply being present with whatever arises in our experience, without directing attention to a specific object or focus. It is a practice of open and spacious awareness, where thoughts, emotions, sounds, and sensations are observed without getting caught up in them. Open awareness meditation cultivates a deep sense of presence, clarity, and expanded consciousness.

Benefits of Meditation and Mindfulness Practices:

Stress Reduction: Meditation and mindfulness practices have been scientifically proven to reduce stress by activating the relaxation response and lowering levels of stress hormones. Regular practice can lead to improved resilience to stressors and increased overall well-being.

Improved Mental Clarity: Meditation and mindfulness practices enhance mental clarity by training the mind to focus and sustain attention. They help quiet the mind, reduce mental chatter, and improve cognitive abilities such as concentration, memory, and problem-solving.

Emotional Balance: These practices cultivate emotional balance by increasing self-awareness and enhancing our capacity to observe and regulate our emotions. They promote a greater understanding of the mind-emotion connection and facilitate a more skillful response to challenging emotions.

Increased Self-Awareness: Meditation and mindfulness practices deepen self-awareness by allowing us to observe our thoughts, emotions, and sensations with non-judgmental awareness. This self-reflective process enhances our understanding of ourselves and supports personal growth and transformation.

Enhanced Well-being: Regular meditation and mindfulness practice have been associated with increased overall well-being, including improved mood, greater life satisfaction, and a heightened sense of inner peace and contentment.

Better Health: Meditation and mindfulness practices have been linked to various physical health benefits, including reduced blood pressure, improved immune function, and enhanced sleep quality. They promote a mind-body connection that supports overall health and vitality.

Spiritual Growth: In the context of the Sattvic teachings, meditation and mindfulness practices are considered pathways to spiritual growth and self-realization. They facilitate a deeper connection with our innermost being, higher consciousness, and the divine.

Incorporating Meditation and Mindfulness into Daily Life:

To fully benefit from meditation and mindfulness practices, it is important to integrate them into our daily lives. Here are some tips to incorporate these practices into your routine:

Consistency: Set aside a specific time each day for your meditation practice. Consistency is key to experiencing the cumulative benefits of these practices.

Start Small: Begin with shorter meditation sessions and gradually increase the duration as you become more comfortable. Even a few minutes of regular practice can make a difference.

Create a Sacred Space: Designate a quiet and comfortable space for your meditation practice. This can be a corner in your home or any place where you feel calm and undisturbed.

Make it a Habit: Integrate meditation and mindfulness into your daily routine by making it a habit. Just as you brush your teeth daily, consider meditation as a non-negotiable part of your self-care routine.

Seek Guidance: If you are new to meditation, consider seeking guidance from experienced teachers or using meditation apps that provide guided meditations. They can provide structure and support as you develop your practice.

Integrate Mindfulness into Daily Activities: Extend the practice of mindfulness beyond formal meditation sessions by bringing mindful awareness to daily activities such as eating, walking, or engaging in conversations. This cultivates a sense of presence and mindfulness throughout the day.

Explore Different Techniques: Experiment with various meditation and mindfulness techniques to find what resonates with you. There are different styles, traditions, and approaches to choose from, so explore and find what suits your needs and preferences.

Practice Self-Compassion: Be gentle and patient with yourself. Meditation is a journey, and your practice will evolve over time. Embrace the ups and downs without judgment or attachment to expectations.

By incorporating meditation and mindfulness practices into our lives, we can experience the numerous benefits they offer. These practices provide us with the tools to cultivate mental clarity, emotional balance, and a deeper connection with ourselves and the world around us. They are powerful pathways to inner peace, self-discovery, and spiritual growth.

A Simple and Balanced Meditation Technique That You Can Practice

Find a comfortable posture: Sit in a comfortable position, either cross-legged on the floor or on a chair with your feet flat on the ground. Ensure that your spine is upright but relaxed, allowing for easy breathing.

Relax your body: Close your eyes gently and take a few deep breaths to relax your body. Allow any tension or tightness to dissolve with each exhale.

Bring attention to your breath: Shift your focus to your breath. Notice the natural flow of your breath as it enters and leaves your body. Feel the sensation of the breath as it moves in and out of your nostrils or the rising and falling of your abdomen.

Be present in the moment: Gently redirect your attention whenever your mind starts to wander. Notice any thoughts, emotions, or sensations that arise, but avoid getting caught up in them. Simply acknowledge their presence and let them go, gently bringing your attention back to the breath.

Cultivate a sense of balance: As you continue to observe your breath, bring your awareness to the balance between inhalation and exhalation. Notice the rhythm and the pause in between each breath. Allow yourself to experience the natural harmony and equilibrium of your breath, symbolizing the balance within you.

Cultivate feelings of calm and peace: With each inhalation, visualize yourself inhaling calmness, clarity, and peace. Imagine these qualities filling your body and mind, cleansing any tension or restlessness. As you exhale, visualize releasing any stress, worries, or negative emotions, allowing them to dissolve and disperse.

Stay present for a few minutes: Continue this practice for a few minutes, maintaining your focus on the breath and the sensations of calm and peace. If your mind wanders, gently bring it back to the breath and the visualization.

Gradual transition: When you feel ready to end the meditation, take a few deep breaths, gradually bring your awareness back to your surroundings, and open your eyes. Take a moment to appreciate the sense of calm and peace you have cultivated.

Remember, meditation is a practice, and it may take time to fully experience its benefits. Start with shorter sessions and gradually increase the duration as you become more comfortable. Consistency and patience are key. Over time, this simple meditation technique can help you cultivate a sense of balance, calm, and peace in your life

2.3 BREATHING TECHNIQUES FOR MENTAL AND EMOTIONAL WELL-BEING

The breath is a powerful tool that can significantly impact our mental and emotional well-being. Various breathing techniques have been developed and practiced for centuries as a means to calm the mind, reduce stress, and promote overall well-being. By consciously directing our breath, we can influence our nervous system, regulate our emotions, and cultivate a sense of inner peace. Let's explore some popular breathing techniques and their benefits:

Deep Abdominal Breathing:

Deep abdominal breathing, also known as diaphragmatic breathing or belly breathing, involves consciously using the diaphragm to take slow, deep breaths. This technique engages the diaphragm muscle, allowing the lungs to fully expand and oxygenate the body. Deep abdominal breathing triggers the body's relaxation response, activating the parasympathetic nervous system, and reducing the physiological effects of stress. It promotes a sense of calm, decreases heart rate and blood pressure, and helps to relieve anxiety and tension.

Box Breathing:

Box breathing, also known as square breathing, is a simple technique that involves equalizing the length of the inhalation, retention, exhalation, and the pause between breaths. It follows a four-count pattern, typically inhaling for a count of four, holding the breath for a count of four, exhaling for a count of four, and holding the breath out for a count of four. Box breathing helps to regulate the breath, induce relaxation, and promote mental clarity and focus. It can be used as a grounding practice in moments of stress or as a regular practice for overall well-being.

Alternate Nostril Breathing:

Alternate nostril breathing, or Nadi Shodhana Pranayama, is a yogic breathing technique that involves alternating the breath between the left and right nostrils. By using the fingers to close one nostril at a time, the breath is directed through each nostril in a rhythmic pattern. This technique balances the flow of energy in the body, harmonizes the left and right hemispheres of the brain, and promotes a sense of balance and harmony. Alternate nostril breathing helps to calm the mind, reduce anxiety, enhance focus, and balance the nervous system.

Ujjayi Breathing:

Ujjayi breathing is a technique commonly used in yoga practice. It involves breathing in and out through the nostrils while slightly constricting the back of the throat, creating a gentle hissing or ocean-like sound. Ujjayi breathing is often referred to as "Victorious Breath" as it promotes a sense of victory over the fluctuations of the mind. It helps to deepen the breath, increase oxygen intake, and calm the nervous system. Ujjayi breathing can be practiced during yoga asanas (poses) or as a standalone technique for relaxation and stress reduction.

4-7-8 Breathing:

The 4-7-8 breathing technique, developed by Dr. Andrew Weil, is a simple and effective method for inducing relaxation and calming the mind. It involves inhaling deeply through the nose for a count of four, holding the breath for a count of seven, and exhaling slowly through the mouth for a count of eight. This pattern is repeated for several cycles. The extended exhalation in the 4-7-8 breathing technique activates the body's relaxation response and helps to slow down the heart rate. It promotes a deep sense of relaxation, reduces anxiety, and can aid in falling asleep.

Kapalabhati Breathing:

Kapalabhati, also known as "Skull Shining Breath," is a dynamic breathing technique originating from the yogic tradition. It involves forceful exhalations through the nose while keeping the inhalation passive and gentle. The exhalations are quick, powerful, and generated from the lower belly. Kapalabhati breathing energizes the body, clears the mind, and helps to release stagnant energy and toxins. It is believed to improve mental clarity, invigorate the nervous system, and enhance overall vitality.

Benefits of Breathing Techniques for Mental and Emotional Well-being:

Stress Reduction: Practicing conscious breathing techniques activates the relaxation response, reduces the production of stress hormones, and calms the nervous system. This leads to a reduction in stress levels, promoting a sense of relaxation and overall well-being.

Emotional Regulation: Breathing techniques help to regulate emotions by activating the parasympathetic nervous system, which is responsible for the "rest and digest" response. By consciously controlling the breath, we can influence our emotional state, promoting feelings of calm, stability, and emotional balance.

Improved Focus and Clarity: Deep, rhythmic breathing increases oxygen flow to the brain, improving cognitive function, focus, and mental clarity. By directing our breath, we can quiet the mind, reduce mental chatter, and enhance our ability to concentrate and make decisions.

Enhanced Energy and Vitality: Certain breathing techniques, such as Kapalabhati, stimulate the nervous system and increase the supply of oxygen to the body and brain. This leads to increased energy levels, improved vitality, and a greater sense of aliveness.

Mind-Body Connection: Breathing techniques deepen the mind-body connection by bringing our awareness to the present moment and the sensations of the breath. This cultivates mindfulness and helps us develop a greater understanding of the subtle interplay between our thoughts, emotions, and physical sensations.

Incorporating Breathing Techniques into Daily Life:

To incorporate breathing techniques into your daily life for mental and emotional well-being, consider the following tips:

Start with Awareness: Begin by simply observing your natural breath without trying to control or manipulate it. Notice the quality, depth, and rhythm of your breath as it flows in and out of your body.

Choose a Technique: Explore different breathing techniques and choose one that resonates with you. Experiment with different techniques to find what feels comfortable and effective for you.

Set Aside Time: Set aside a few minutes each day to practice your chosen breathing technique. It can be in the morning to start your day with calmness or in the evening to unwind and relax.

Integrate Throughout the Day: Incorporate conscious breathing into your daily activities. Take a few moments to pause and take deep breaths during moments of stress, before important tasks, or when you need to refocus and re-energize.

Practice Mindful Breathing: Cultivate mindfulness by bringing your attention to the sensations of your breath throughout the day. Notice the feeling of air entering and leaving your nostrils, the rise and fall of your abdomen, or the expansion and contraction of your chest.

Find Support: Consider attending a breathing workshop, joining a yoga class, or using mobile apps that provide guided breathing exercises. These resources can offer guidance, inspiration, and support as you explore and deepen your breathing practice.

Remember, breathing techniques are gentle and safe practices that can be adapted to suit your individual needs. Consistent practice is key to experiencing the benefits, so commit to incorporating these techniques into your daily routine. With time and dedication, you can harness the power of your breath to enhance your mental and emotional well-being.

3.THE SATTVIC DIET IN PRACTICE: NOURISHING THE BODY

The Sattvic diet is rooted in the principles of Ayurveda, an ancient Indian system of medicine and holistic living. It emphasizes the consumption of pure, fresh, and natural foods to promote physical health, mental clarity, and spiritual well-being. The Sattvic diet is considered to be the purest and most harmonious diet, designed to support the body's natural balance and nourish the mind and spirit. Let's explore the key aspects and benefits of the Sattvic diet in practice:

Focus on Pure and Whole Foods:

The Sattvic diet emphasizes the consumption of pure, unprocessed, and whole foods. It encourages the consumption of fresh fruits, vegetables, whole grains, nuts, seeds, legumes, and dairy products that are obtained from ethical and sustainable sources. These foods are considered to be full of life-force energy (prana) and are believed to promote vitality, clarity, and overall well-being.

Plant-Based Emphasis:

The Sattvic diet places a strong emphasis on plant-based foods.

Fresh fruits and vegetables are rich in vitamins, minerals, antioxidants, and fiber, providing essential nutrients for optimal health. They are easily digestible, alkalizing, and help to cleanse and detoxify the body. Consuming a variety of seasonal and locally grown produce is encouraged to support the body's natural rhythms.

Satvik Foods:

Certain foods are considered Sattvic and are believed to promote purity, clarity, and spiritual growth. These include fresh fruits, vegetables, whole grains (such as brown rice, quinoa, and millet), legumes (such as lentils and chickpeas), nuts and seeds, dairy products (such as milk, ghee, and paneer), honey, and herbal teas. These foods are believed to be light, easy to digest, and free from toxins, promoting physical and mental balance.

Mindful Preparation and Cooking:

The Sattvic diet emphasizes the importance of mindful preparation and cooking. Foods should be prepared and cooked with love, care, and positive intentions. Avoiding overcooking, excessive use of spices, and processed ingredients is encouraged. Gentle cooking methods, such as steaming, boiling, sautéing, or baking, help to preserve the nutritional integrity of the foods.

Moderation and Balance:

The Sattvic diet promotes a sense of moderation and balance in eating. It encourages mindful eating, listening to the body's hunger and fullness cues, and avoiding overeating. Eating slowly, chewing food thoroughly, and savoring each bite promotes better digestion and assimilation of nutrients. It is also recommended to eat regular meals and maintain a consistent eating schedule to support the body's natural rhythms.

Hydration:

Proper hydration is vital for overall health and well-being. Drinking pure and filtered water is encouraged in the Sattvic diet to maintain hydration, flush out toxins, and support various bodily functions. Herbal teas, especially those made from Ayurvedic herbs like tulsi (holy basil), chamomile, or ginger, can also be consumed to promote digestion and balance.

Benefits of the Sattvic Diet:

Physical Well-being: The Sattvic diet provides the body with a wide range of essential nutrients, vitamins, and minerals from fresh, whole foods. It supports optimal digestion, improves energy levels, strengthens the immune system, and promotes overall physical health.

Mental Clarity: The purity and lightness of Sattvic foods are believed to promote mental clarity, focus, and concentration. It is thought to calm the mind, reduce mental and emotional turbulence, and enhance cognitive function.

Emotional Balance: The Sattvic diet emphasizes foods that are believed to have a calming and balancing effect on the mind and emotions. By avoiding heavy, processed, and stimulating foods, it can help stabilize mood, reduce anxiety, and promote emotional well-being.

Spiritual Growth: The Sattvic diet is seen as a tool for spiritual growth and self-realization. It is believed that consuming pure, natural foods enhances spiritual awareness, intuition, and connection to higher consciousness. It supports the practice of meditation and other spiritual practices by promoting clarity and purity of mind.

Incorporating the Sattvic Diet into Your Life:

Gradual Transition: Transitioning to a Sattvic diet can be done gradually. Start by incorporating more fresh fruits, vegetables, whole grains, and plant-based proteins into your meals. Reduce or eliminate processed foods, refined sugars, and excessive spices.

Mindful Eating: Practice mindful eating by paying attention to the quality of your food, chewing thoroughly, and savoring the flavors and textures. Eat in a calm and peaceful environment, free from distractions.

Seasonal and Local Foods: Emphasize seasonal and locally sourced foods to align with nature's cycles and support the body's needs in different seasons. This ensures freshness, optimal taste, and higher nutritional value.

Self-Awareness: Observe how different foods make you feel physically, mentally, and emotionally. Notice the effects of Sattvic foods on your overall well-being and make adjustments accordingly.

Individual Adaptations: The Sattvic diet can be adapted to individual needs, preferences, and health conditions. Seek guidance from a qualified Ayurvedic practitioner or nutritionist who can provide personalized recommendations.

Remember, the Sattvic diet is not about strict rules or restrictions but rather about cultivating a mindful and conscious approach to food choices. It is a holistic lifestyle that extends beyond diet and incorporates other aspects of well-being such as mindfulness, meditation, and conscious living. By embracing the Sattvic diet, you can nourish your body, promote mental clarity, and align with a more harmonious and balanced way of life.

3.1 UNDERSTANDING SATTVIC FOODS AND THEIR QUALITIES

Sattvic foods are an essential component of the Sattvic diet, which is based on the principles of Ayurveda and emphasizes the consumption of pure, fresh, and natural foods. Sattvic foods are believed to have a harmonizing and purifying effect on the body, mind, and spirit. They are considered to be light, nourishing, and promote clarity, balance, and spiritual growth. Let's explore the key qualities and examples of Sattvic foods:

Purity:

Sattvic foods are pure and free from toxins, chemicals, and additives. They are obtained from ethical and sustainable sources, such as organic farms or local farmers' markets. These foods are believed to be filled with life-force energy (prana) and promote vitality and overall well-being.

Examples: Fresh fruits, vegetables, whole grains, nuts, seeds, legumes, dairy products (from ethical sources), honey, herbal teas.

Lightness:

Sattvic foods are light and easily digestible. They do not burden the digestive system and promote optimal digestion and assimilation of nutrients. Lightness in food helps to maintain clarity of mind and prevents lethargy or heaviness after meals.

Examples: Fresh fruits (such as apples, pears, berries, melons), leafy greens (such as spinach, kale, lettuce), steamed vegetables, whole grains (such as brown rice, quinoa, amaranth), lentils, mung beans, almonds.

Freshness:

Sattvic foods are consumed in their natural, fresh, and seasonal form. Fresh foods are believed to be higher in prana and retain their nutritional value. They are also more vibrant in taste, texture, and aroma.

Examples: Fresh fruits, seasonal vegetables, herbs, sprouts, freshly made juices, freshly prepared meals.

Vitality:

Sattvic foods are vibrant and full of vitality. They are rich in essential nutrients, vitamins, minerals, and antioxidants that support optimal health and well-being. Vitality in food helps to nourish the body, increase energy levels, and promote overall vitality.

Examples: Fresh fruits (such as oranges, mangoes, bananas), leafy greens (such as spinach, kale, chard), sprouts, almonds, sunflower seeds, coconut.

Sattvic Flavors:

Sattvic foods are naturally flavorful and often have a sweet, sour, or astringent taste. These flavors are believed to promote balance, satisfaction, and a sense of grounding.

Examples: Sweet fruits (such as dates, figs, grapes), ripe mangoes, lemons, unsweetened yogurt, ghee (clarified butter), almonds, sesame seeds.

Mind-Body Connection:

Sattvic foods are known to promote a strong mind-body connection. They are believed to support mental clarity, enhance focus, and calm the mind. Consuming Sattvic foods is seen as a way to cultivate inner peace and harmony.

Examples: Herbal teas (such as chamomile, lavender, tulsi), almonds, walnuts, raisins, ghee, whole grains.

Benefits of Sattvic Foods:

Mental Clarity: Sattvic foods support mental clarity and focus. They are believed to calm the mind, reduce mental and emotional turbulence, and enhance cognitive function.

Emotional Balance: Sattvic foods help to promote emotional balance and stability. They are believed to have a calming effect on the nervous system, reduce anxiety, and support a positive emotional state.

Physical Well-being: Sattvic foods provide essential nutrients, vitamins, and minerals, promoting overall physical health. They support optimal digestion, boost the immune system, and provide sustained energy.

Spiritual Growth: Sattvic foods are considered conducive to spiritual growth and self-realization. They are believed to enhance spiritual awareness, promote purity of mind, and facilitate a deeper connection to higher consciousness.

Incorporating Sattvic Foods into Your Diet:

Choose Fresh and Seasonal Foods: Opt for fresh, seasonal fruits, vegetables, and herbs. These foods are abundant in nutrients and prana, and their flavors are enhanced.

Emphasize Whole Grains: Include whole grains like brown rice, quinoa, amaranth, and millet in your meals. They provide sustained energy and are rich in fiber and essential nutrients.

Include Plant-based Proteins: Incorporate plant-based proteins like lentils, mung beans, chickpeas, and tofu. These foods are nutrient-dense and support muscle growth and repair.

Prioritize Fresh Fruits and Vegetables: Consume a variety of fresh fruits and vegetables daily. Include a rainbow of colors to ensure a wide range of nutrients and antioxidants.

Enjoy Nuts and Seeds: Include almonds, walnuts, sunflower seeds, sesame seeds, and pumpkin seeds in your diet. They are rich in healthy fats, protein, and essential minerals.

Use Healthy Cooking Methods: Opt for cooking methods such as steaming, sautéing, or baking to retain the nutritional value and flavors of the ingredients.

Mindful Eating: Practice mindful eating by savoring each bite, chewing thoroughly, and eating in a calm and peaceful environment.

Remember, the Sattvic diet is a flexible and individualized approach. Listen to your body's needs and adjust the quantities and combinations of foods according to your own constitution and preferences. Incorporating Sattvic foods into your diet can promote nourishment, balance, and overall well-being.

3.2 PLANNING A BALANCED SATTVIC MEAL

Planning a Balanced Sattvic Meal

When following the Sattvic diet, it is important to plan and prepare balanced meals that nourish the body, mind, and spirit. A balanced Sattvic meal incorporates a variety of fresh, whole foods, ensures adequate nutrients, and promotes optimal digestion. Here are some key principles and guidelines to consider when planning a balanced Sattvic meal:

Include All Food Groups:

A balanced Sattvic meal should include foods from all major food groups to ensure a wide range of nutrients. These food groups include:

a. Whole Grains: Choose whole grains such as brown rice, quinoa, millet, or amaranth. These grains are rich in fiber, essential minerals, and complex carbohydrates.

b. Fresh Fruits and Vegetables: Incorporate a variety of fresh, seasonal fruits and vegetables. They provide essential vitamins, minerals, antioxidants, and fiber.

c. Legumes and Plant-based Proteins: Include legumes like lentils, mung beans, chickpeas, or tofu. These plant-based proteins are rich in essential amino acids.

d. Nuts and Seeds: Add a handful of almonds, walnuts, sunflower seeds, sesame seeds, or pumpkin seeds. They provide healthy fats, protein, and essential minerals.

e. Dairy Products (if desired): Include dairy products like milk, ghee (clarified butter), or yogurt if you consume them. Choose organic and ethically sourced options.

f. Herbal Teas: Finish your meal with a calming herbal tea, such as chamomile, tulsi (holy basil), or ginger tea. These teas aid digestion and promote relaxation.

Balance the Six Tastes:

According to Ayurveda, it is important to incorporate all six tastes into each meal to ensure satisfaction and balance. The six tastes are sweet, sour, salty, bitter, pungent, and astringent. Here's how you can include them in a Sattvic meal:

a. Sweet: Include naturally sweet foods like ripe fruits, dates, honey, or sweet vegetables like carrots and sweet potatoes.

b. Sour: Add a touch of sourness with lemon or lime juice, a sprinkle of raw mango powder (amchur), or fermented foods like yogurt or pickles.

c. Salty: Use a small amount of natural salts like Himalayan pink salt or sea salt to enhance flavors. Be mindful of the quantity and avoid excessive salt intake.

d. Bitter: Incorporate bitter greens like kale, dandelion greens, or arugula. You can also include bitter herbs like fenugreek or turmeric.

e. Pungent: Add a touch of heat with spices like ginger, black pepper, cayenne pepper, or mustard seeds. These spices aid digestion and add flavor.

f. Astringent: Include astringent foods like legumes, lentils, and some vegetables such as broccoli or cauliflower. They help balance excess moisture in the body.

Mindful Portions:

Practice mindful eating and portion control to avoid overeating and maintain a light and balanced meal. Listen to your body's hunger and fullness cues and eat until you are comfortably satisfied. Avoid excessive consumption of heavy or processed foods.

Cooking Methods:

Choose gentle cooking methods that preserve the nutritional value of the ingredients. Steaming, boiling, sautéing, or baking are preferred over deep-frying or heavy frying methods. These methods help retain the natural flavors and qualities of the ingredients.

Fresh and Seasonal Ingredients:

Prioritize fresh and seasonal ingredients in your meal planning. Fresh foods are believed to be higher in prana (life-force energy) and offer optimal taste and nutritional value. They are also in harmony with nature's cycles.

Hydration:

Include hydrating elements in your meal, such as water-rich fruits, herbal teas, or infused water. Staying adequately hydrated supports digestion, detoxification, and overall well-being.

Mindful Preparation:

Prepare your meals with love, mindfulness, and positive intentions. Engage in the cooking process as a meditative practice, being fully present and appreciating the nourishment it provides.

3.3 INCORPORATING SEASONAL AND ORGANIC FOODS

One of the key principles of the Sattvic diet is the emphasis on consuming seasonal and organic foods. This approach aligns with the natural rhythms of the Earth and promotes optimal health, vitality, and environmental sustainability. Let's explore the benefits and strategies for incorporating seasonal and organic foods into your Sattvic lifestyle:

Benefits of Seasonal Foods:

Nutritional Value: Seasonal foods are harvested at their peak ripeness and offer higher nutritional value compared to out-of-season produce. They are rich in essential vitamins, minerals, antioxidants, and phytonutrients that support overall health and well-being.

Flavor and Taste: Seasonal foods are known for their superior flavor and taste. They are fresh, vibrant, and offer a more enjoyable culinary experience. Eating in alignment with the seasons allows you to savor the unique flavors each season has to offer.

Environmental Sustainability: Choosing seasonal foods helps reduce the carbon footprint associated with long-distance transportation and storage of out-of-season produce. It supports local farmers and promotes sustainable agricultural practices.

Cost-Effectiveness: Seasonal foods are often more affordable due to their abundance during their peak harvest. By choosing seasonal produce, you can save money on your grocery bills while enjoying high-quality, nutritious foods.

Tips for Incorporating Seasonal Foods:

Know Your Seasons: Familiarize yourself with the seasonal produce in your region. Research local farmers' markets, join community-supported agriculture (CSA) programs, or consult seasonal produce guides specific to your area.

Shop at Farmers' Markets: Visit farmers' markets to find a wide variety of locally grown, seasonal produce. It's an excellent opportunity to connect with local farmers, learn about their farming practices, and support your community.

Join a CSA Program: Community-supported agriculture (CSA) programs allow you to receive a weekly or monthly share of fresh, seasonal produce directly from local farms. It's a convenient way to enjoy a diverse range of seasonal foods and support local agriculture.

Grow Your Own: Consider starting a small garden or growing herbs and vegetables in pots or raised beds. This allows you to cultivate your own seasonal produce and reconnect with the natural cycles of growth and harvest.

Benefits of Organic Foods:

Reduced Exposure to Chemicals: Organic foods are grown without the use of synthetic fertilizers, pesticides, herbicides, or genetically modified organisms (GMOs). Choosing organic reduces your exposure to potentially harmful chemicals and promotes overall health.

Higher Nutritional Content: Organic farming practices prioritize soil health, which leads to nutrient-rich crops. Organic foods often contain higher levels of beneficial nutrients such as vitamins, minerals, and antioxidants.

Environmental Conservation: Organic farming methods focus on sustainability and biodiversity. They promote soil health, water conservation, and the preservation of beneficial insects and wildlife. Choosing organic supports eco-friendly agricultural practices and contributes to a healthier planet.

Support for Small-Scale Farmers: Organic farming often involves smaller-scale operations that prioritize sustainable and ethical practices. By purchasing organic foods, you support local farmers and contribute to the growth of organic farming communities.

Tips for Incorporating Organic Foods:

Read Labels: Look for the USDA Organic label or other trusted organic certifications when purchasing packaged or processed foods. This ensures that the product meets organic standards.

Choose Local Organic: Seek out local organic farms or suppliers in your area. Local farmer's markets, co-ops, or organic grocery stores are excellent places to find a variety of organic produce and other food products.

Grow Your Own: Consider starting an organic garden at home. This allows you to have control over the quality of the soil and the use of pesticides, ensuring that your homegrown produce is organic and fresh.

Prioritize Key Organic Foods: If buying all organic is not feasible, prioritize purchasing organic versions of foods known to have higher pesticide residue levels, such as strawberries, spinach, apples, and bell peppers.

By incorporating seasonal and organic foods into your Sattvic diet, you can enhance the freshness, flavor, and nutritional value of your meals. It also fosters a deeper connection with nature, promotes sustainable practices, and supports local farmers. Remember to choose wisely, listen to your body's needs, and enjoy the abundance of wholesome foods nature provides each season.

3.4 Sattvic Cooking Methods and Recipes

In the Sattvic diet, the way food is prepared is as important as the ingredients themselves. Sattvic cooking methods prioritize simplicity, freshness, and the preservation of natural flavors and nutrients. Let's explore some commonly used Sattvic cooking methods and discover a few delicious Sattvic recipes:

Steaming: Steaming is a gentle cooking method that helps retain the natural flavors, colors, and nutrients of the ingredients. It involves using steam to cook food without submerging it in water or exposing it to direct heat. Steaming vegetables, grains, and legumes is a popular Sattvic cooking technique.

Recipe Idea: Steamed Vegetable Medley

Ingredients:

Assorted vegetables (carrots, broccoli, cauliflower, zucchini, etc.)

Fresh herbs (such as basil or cilantro)

Lemon juice

Salt and pepper to taste

Instructions:

Chop the vegetables into bite-sized pieces.

Place a steamer basket or colander over a pot of boiling water.

Add the vegetables to the steamer basket and cover with a lid.

Steam the vegetables for 5-10 minutes or until they are tender but still crisp.

Transfer the steamed vegetables to a serving dish and toss with fresh herbs, lemon juice, salt, and pepper. Serve hot.

Sautéing: Sautéing involves cooking food quickly in a small amount of oil or ghee over medium-high heat. It helps to preserve the flavors and textures of the ingredients while adding a touch of richness.

Recipe Idea: Sautéed Greens with Garlic

Ingredients:

Assorted leafy greens (spinach, kale, Swiss chard, etc.)

Garlic cloves, minced

Ghee or olive oil

Salt and pepper to taste

Instructions:

Wash the greens thoroughly and remove any tough stems.

Heat ghee or olive oil in a pan over medium heat.

Add minced garlic and sauté for a minute until fragrant.

Add the greens to the pan and sauté until wilted but still vibrant green.

Season with salt and pepper to taste.

Serve as a side dish or as a base for other Sattvic recipes.

Baking: Baking is a versatile cooking method that allows for the creation of a wide range of Sattvic dishes. It involves cooking food in an oven using dry heat, often without added fats or oils. Baking helps to concentrate flavors and create delicious, nourishing meals.

Recipe Idea: Baked Sweet Potatoes with Tahini Drizzle

Ingredients:

Sweet potatoes

Tahini

Lemon juice

Fresh parsley, chopped

Salt and pepper to taste

Instructions:

Preheat the oven to 400°F (200°C).

Wash sweet potatoes thoroughly and pierce them with a fork.

Place the sweet potatoes on a baking sheet and bake for 45-60 minutes, or until they are soft and cooked through.

In a small bowl, whisk together tahini, lemon juice, chopped parsley, salt, and pepper to make the drizzle.

Once the sweet potatoes are cooked, slice them lengthwise and drizzle with the tahini mixture.

Serve as a nourishing and satisfying Sattvic meal.

Raw Preparations: Raw food preparations are an integral part of the Sattvic diet. Consuming raw fruits, vegetables, and salads helps to preserve their natural enzymes, vitamins, and antioxidants.

Recipe Idea: Fresh Fruit Salad

Ingredients:

Assorted seasonal fruits (such as mangoes, berries, melons, etc.)

Fresh mint leaves, chopped

Lime or lemon juice

Instructions:

Wash and cut the fruits into bite-sized pieces.

Combine the fruits in a bowl and toss gently.

Sprinkle with fresh mint leaves and drizzle with lime or lemon juice.

Allow the flavors to meld for a few minutes before serving.

Enjoy the refreshing and energizing flavors of this Sattvic fruit salad.

These are just a few examples of Sattvic cooking methods and recipes. The key is to prioritize simplicity, freshness, and the use of high-quality ingredients. Experiment with different combinations of vegetables, grains, legumes, and spices to create nourishing and balanced Sattvic meals. Enjoy the process of cooking mindfully and savor the flavors of each ingredient as you embrace the Sattvic lifestyle.

4.THE HEALING POWER OF SATTVIC HERBS AND SPICES

In the Sattvic diet, herbs and spices play a vital role in enhancing the flavors of meals while providing numerous health benefits. Sattvic herbs and spices are valued not only for their taste but also for their therapeutic properties that promote overall well-being. Let's explore some commonly used Sattvic herbs and spices and their healing benefits:

Turmeric (Curcuma longa):

Turmeric is a vibrant yellow spice commonly used in Sattvic cooking. It contains a powerful compound called curcumin, known for its anti-inflammatory and antioxidant properties. Turmeric supports digestion, enhances immune function, and promotes healthy skin. It is often used in curries, soups, and rice dishes.

Cumin (Cuminum cyminum):

Cumin seeds have a warm and earthy flavor. They aid in digestion, help alleviate bloating and gas, and promote healthy metabolism. Cumin is commonly used in Sattvic recipes such as dals (lentil soups), vegetable dishes, and spice blends.

Coriander (Coriandrum sativum):

Coriander is known for its distinct flavor and aroma. It aids in digestion, detoxification, and supports healthy blood sugar levels. Coriander seeds and fresh coriander leaves (cilantro) are commonly used in Sattvic cooking to enhance the flavors of soups, stews, and salads.

Ginger (Zingiber officinale):

Ginger has a warming and spicy flavor. It aids in digestion, reduces inflammation, and boosts the immune system. Ginger can be used fresh, grated, or in powdered form in a variety of Sattvic dishes, including teas, soups, and stir-fries.

Holy Basil (Ocimum tenuiflorum):

Holy Basil, also known as Tulsi, is considered sacred in Indian culture. It has a refreshing and slightly peppery flavor. Holy Basil is known for its adaptogenic properties, reducing stress, promoting mental clarity, and boosting immunity. It can be used in herbal teas, infused water, and as a seasoning for salads and soups.

Cardamom (Elettaria cardamomum):

Cardamom has a sweet and aromatic flavor. It aids digestion, freshens breath, and has a calming effect on the body and mind. Cardamom is often used in desserts, hot beverages, and rice-based dishes in the Sattvic cuisine.

Ashwagandha (Withania somnifera):

Ashwagandha is a powerful adaptogenic herb widely used in Ayurveda. It helps reduce stress, support adrenal health, and promote overall vitality. Ashwagandha can be consumed in powdered form or added to warm milk or herbal teas.

Brahmi (Bacopa monnieri):

Brahmi is a renowned herb for its cognitive-enhancing properties. It supports mental clarity, memory, and concentration. Brahmi can be consumed as a herbal supplement or added to drinks like smoothies or infused water.

Fennel (Foeniculum vulgare):

Fennel seeds have a licorice-like flavor and are known for their digestive properties. They help alleviate bloating, support healthy digestion, and freshen breath. Fennel seeds can be chewed after meals or used in spice blends for added flavor.

Saffron (Crocus sativus):

Saffron is a prized spice known for its vibrant color and delicate flavor. It is considered uplifting and is used to promote relaxation, improve mood, and support emotional well-being. Saffron is often used in desserts, milk-based beverages, and rice dishes.

When incorporating herbs and spices into your Sattvic diet, choose high-quality organic sources whenever possible. Experiment with different combinations to enhance the flavors and therapeutic benefits of your meals. Remember to use herbs and spices in moderation and according to your body's needs and sensitivities.

The healing power of Sattvic herbs and spices goes beyond their culinary value. They provide a natural way to support your overall health and well-being, contributing to the holistic harmony of the body, mind, and spirit.

4.1 AYURVEDIC PERSPECTIVE ON HERBS AND SPICES

In Ayurveda, an ancient system of medicine originating from India, herbs and spices play a crucial role in promoting health, balance, and well-being. Ayurveda recognizes the unique properties of herbs and spices and their ability to influence the body, mind, and spirit. Let's delve into the Ayurvedic perspective on herbs and spices and explore their therapeutic benefits:

The Three Doshas:

According to Ayurveda, every individual has a unique constitution or dosha, which is determined by the balance of the three fundamental energies—Vata, Pitta, and Kapha. Herbs and spices are categorized based on their taste (rasa), heating or cooling effect (virya), and post-digestive effect (vipaka), and their impact on the doshas.

Vata-Pacifying Herbs and Spices: Herbs and spices with sweet, sour, and salty tastes help balance the Vata dosha, which governs movement and communication in the body. Examples include ginger, cinnamon, cardamom, fennel, and ashwagandha.

Pitta-Pacifying Herbs and Spices: Cooling herbs and spices with bitter, sweet, and astringent tastes help balance the Pitta dosha, responsible for digestion, metabolism, and transformation. Examples include coriander, cilantro, turmeric, fennel, and

Brahmi.

Kapha-Pacifying Herbs and Spices: Warming and stimulating herbs and spices with pungent, bitter, and astringent tastes help balance the Kapha dosha, which governs stability and structure in the body. Examples include black pepper, ginger, cinnamon, clove, and holy basil.

Healing Properties:

Ayurvedic texts describe the medicinal properties of various herbs and spices. They are classified based on their actions, such as promoting digestion, reducing inflammation, improving immunity, supporting detoxification, calming the mind, and balancing specific organs or body systems.

Digestive Herbs and Spices: Herbs and spices like ginger, cumin, coriander, and fennel aid digestion, stimulate appetite, reduce bloating, and alleviate indigestion.

Anti-inflammatory Herbs and Spices: Turmeric, ginger, cinnamon, and coriander possess anti-inflammatory properties, helping to reduce inflammation in the body and support joint health.

Immune-Boosting Herbs and Spices: Holy basil, ashwagandha, turmeric, and ginger are known to enhance immune function, improve resilience to stress, and support overall vitality.

Nervine Herbs and Spices: Brahmi, ashwagandha, cardamom, and holy basil are considered nervine herbs, supporting the nervous system, promoting mental clarity, and reducing stress and anxiety.

Ayurvedic Formulations:

In Ayurveda, herbs and spices are often combined in specific formulations to enhance their efficacy and create a synergistic effect. These formulations, known as churnas, teas, herbal blends, or Ayurvedic medicines, are tailored to address specific imbalances or health conditions.

Triphala: A popular Ayurvedic formulation consisting of three fruits—amalaki (Indian gooseberry), bibhitaki, and haritaki. Triphala supports digestion, detoxification, and elimination.

Chyawanprash: A potent herbal jam containing a blend of herbs, spices, and amla (Indian gooseberry). Chyawanprash is known for its rejuvenating and immune-enhancing properties.

Herbal Teas: Ayurvedic herbal teas, such as ginger tea, tulsi tea (holy basil), and cumin coriander fennel tea (CCF tea), are commonly consumed to support digestion, promote relaxation, and balance the doshas.

Individualized Approach:

Ayurveda recognizes that each person is unique, and the effects of herbs and spices may vary based on an individual's constitution, imbalances, and specific health conditions. Ayurvedic practitioners assess the person's dosha imbalance and consider factors such as age, season, and digestive strength to create a personalized herbal protocol.

It is essential to consult with a qualified Ayurvedic practitioner or healthcare provider before incorporating herbs and spices into your routine to ensure their suitability for your specific needs.

In conclusion, Ayurveda views herbs and spices as powerful tools for maintaining health and restoring balance in the body and mind. Understanding the properties and effects of herbs and spices from an Ayurvedic perspective can help you make informed choices in selecting and using them to support your overall well-being.

4.2 SATTVIC HERBS FOR ENHANCING WELL-BEING

Sattvic herbs are an integral part of the Sattvic lifestyle and are valued for their ability to promote physical, mental, and spiritual well-being. These herbs possess qualities that align with the Sattvic principles of purity, clarity, and balance. Let's explore some commonly used Sattvic herbs and their benefits:

Tulsi (Holy Basil):

Tulsi, also known as Holy Basil, is considered a sacred herb in Ayurveda. It has a refreshing and slightly peppery flavor. Tulsi is known for its adaptogenic properties, which help the body adapt to stress and promote overall well-being. It supports the immune system, calms the mind, and enhances clarity and focus. Tulsi can be consumed as herbal tea or added to dishes as a seasoning.

Ashwagandha:

Ashwagandha is a powerful adaptogenic herb that has been used for centuries in Ayurveda. It helps the body adapt to stress, supports adrenal health, and promotes physical and mental vitality. Ashwagandha is known for its calming effect on the nervous system, aiding in relaxation and sleep. It can be consumed as a powdered supplement, infused in warm milk, or added to smoothies.

Brahmi:

Brahmi, also known as Bacopa monnieri, is a renowned herb for enhancing cognitive function and promoting mental well-being. It supports memory, concentration, and mental clarity. Brahmi is often used in Ayurvedic formulations to calm the mind and reduce anxiety and stress. It can be consumed as a supplement or added to teas and beverages.

Gotu Kola:

Gotu Kola, also known as Centella asiatica, is a herb traditionally used in Ayurveda for its rejuvenating and balancing properties. It supports healthy skin, improves circulation, and enhances mental function. Gotu Kola is considered a brain tonic, supporting cognitive health and promoting a calm and focused mind. It can be consumed as a tea or included in salads and soups.

Shatavari:

Shatavari, also known as Asparagus racemosus, is a revered herb for women's health in Ayurveda. It supports hormonal balance, reproductive health, and promotes vitality. Shatavari is known for its nourishing and cooling properties, helping to balance the Pitta dosha and calm the mind. It can be consumed as a powdered supplement or added to warm milk or teas.

Triphala:

Triphala is a combination of three fruits—amalaki (Indian gooseberry), bibhitaki, and haritaki. It is a potent herbal formula widely used in Ayurveda to support digestion, detoxification, and overall well-being. Triphala helps regulate bowel movements, supports healthy digestion, and provides antioxidant support. It can be consumed as a powdered supplement or infused in warm water or tea.

Licorice (Yashtimadhu):

Licorice, or Yashtimadhu, is a sweet and soothing herb that helps balance the Vata and Pitta doshas. It supports digestive health, soothes the respiratory system, and promotes a healthy throat and voice. Licorice is often used in Ayurvedic formulations to support the body's natural defenses and enhance overall well-being. It can be consumed as a tea or included in herbal blends.

Calamus (Vacha):

Calamus, or Vacha, is an herb known for its stimulating and purifying properties. It supports mental clarity, enhances memory, and promotes focus and concentration. Calamus is often used in Ayurveda to balance the Kapha dosha and improve cognitive function. It can be consumed as a powdered supplement or added to herbal formulations.

It's important to note that individual needs and sensitivities may vary, and it is recommended to consult with an Ayurvedic practitioner or healthcare provider before incorporating Sattvic herbs into your routine. They can provide personalized guidance based on your constitution, imbalances, and specific health concerns.

Incorporating Sattvic herbs into your daily routine can support overall well-being, promote balance, and enhance your Sattvic lifestyle. Experiment with these herbs, and discover the ones that resonate with you, bringing harmony to your body, mind, and spirit.

4.3 PREPARING HERBAL INFUSIONS AND TONICS

Herbal infusions and tonics are popular methods of utilizing the therapeutic properties of herbs for promoting health and well-being. These preparations allow the extraction of beneficial compounds from herbs, creating potent and nourishing beverages. Let's explore the process of preparing herbal infusions and tonics:

Herbal Infusions:

Herbal infusions involve steeping herbs in hot water to extract their medicinal properties. Follow these steps to prepare a herbal infusion:

a. Choose your herbs: Select high-quality dried herbs or a combination of herbs that align with your specific health goals or concerns. Common herbs used in infusions include chamomile, nettle, peppermint, lemon balm, and rose petals.

b. Boil water: Bring filtered water to a boil. The amount of water will depend on the desired strength of the infusion and the number of servings you wish to make.

c. Preparing the herbs: Place the desired amount of dried herbs (usually 1-2 teaspoons per cup of water) in a teapot, infuser, or a heat-resistant container.

d. Pour the hot water: Pour the boiling water over the herbs, ensuring they are fully submerged. Cover the container with a lid or a plate to retain the volatile oils and active compounds.

e. Steeping time: Allow the herbs to steep for around 5-10 minutes, or longer if desired. The steeping time can vary based on the herbs used and your personal preference. Some delicate herbs require shorter steeping times, while others benefit from longer steeping for a more potent infusion.

f. Strain and serve: After steeping, strain the infusion using a fine mesh strainer or a tea infuser. Pour the herbal infusion into cups or mugs and enjoy it warm or chilled. You may sweeten it with honey or add a slice of lemon if desired.

Herbal Tonics:

Herbal tonics are more concentrated preparations that often involve simmering herbs in water to extract their medicinal compounds. Follow these steps to prepare a herbal tonic:

a. Choose your herbs: Select a combination of herbs that support your specific health goals or concerns. Common herbs used in tonics include astragalus, burdock root, dandelion root, ginger, and licorice.

b. Measure and prepare the herbs: Depending on the desired strength and potency, measure the herbs accordingly. You can use a ratio of 1 part herbs to 10 parts water as a general guideline.

c. Simmer the herbs: Place the herbs in a pot and add filtered water. Bring the mixture to a boil, then reduce the heat to a gentle simmer. Allow the herbs to simmer for about 20-30 minutes to extract their beneficial properties.

d. Strain and store: After simmering, remove the pot from the heat and let it cool slightly. Strain the liquid through a fine mesh strainer or cheesecloth to remove the herb particles. Pour the tonic into a glass jar or bottle for storage.

e. Serving and usage: Herbal tonics can be consumed in small amounts daily as a therapeutic tonic. You can drink it as is or dilute it with water or a dash of honey. Store the tonic in the refrigerator and consume within a few days for optimal freshness and potency.

Remember to research and consult with an herbalist or healthcare practitioner to determine the appropriate herbs and dosages for your specific needs. Some herbs may have contraindications or interactions with certain medications or health conditions.

By preparing herbal infusions and tonics, you can harness the healing power of herbs and enjoy their nourishing benefits. These preparations offer a delightful and natural way to support your well-being and integrate herbs into your daily routine.

5.SATTVIC LIFESTYLE PRACTICES FOR HOLISTIC WELLNESS

A Sattvic lifestyle goes beyond just the Sattvic diet and encompasses various practices that promote holistic wellness and balance in the body, mind, and spirit. These practices help create an environment conducive to self-awareness, inner harmony, and overall well-being. Let's explore some key Sattvic lifestyle practices:

Mindful Eating:

In addition to following a Sattvic diet, practicing mindful eating is crucial. This involves being fully present and aware of the food you consume, savoring each bite, and cultivating gratitude for the nourishment it provides. Chew your food thoroughly and eat in a calm and relaxed environment, free from distractions. This practice enhances digestion, promotes mindful awareness of your body's needs, and fosters a deeper connection with your food.

Conscious Movement:

Engaging in conscious movement practices, such as yoga, tai chi, or qigong, helps promote physical health, flexibility, and vitality. These practices incorporate mindful breathing, gentle stretches, and flowing movements that cultivate balance, strength, and inner peace. Regular physical activity not only enhances physical well-being but also supports mental clarity and emotional balance.

Meditation and Breathwork:

Meditation and breathwork are integral practices in the Sattvic lifestyle. Meditation allows you to quiet the mind, cultivate inner stillness, and connect with your true nature. Choose a meditation technique that resonates with you, whether it's focused attention on the breath, mantra repetition, or mindfulness meditation. Practice regularly to experience increased mental clarity, reduced stress, and a deep sense of peace.

Breathwork, such as pranayama in yoga, involves conscious control and regulation of the breath. Techniques like deep belly breathing, alternate nostril breathing, or Kapalabhati can help calm the mind, balance the nervous system, and increase energy flow throughout the body. Incorporating breathwork into your daily routine promotes relaxation, mental focus, and vitality.

Self-Reflection and Journaling:

Engaging in self-reflection and journaling allows you to explore your thoughts, emotions, and experiences, fostering self-awareness and personal growth. Set aside time regularly to reflect on your day, express gratitude, set intentions, and examine any patterns or beliefs that may be hindering your well-being. Journaling can be a cathartic practice that helps release emotions, gain clarity, and cultivate a positive mindset.

Nurturing Relationships:

Cultivating healthy and supportive relationships is an essential aspect of a Sattvic lifestyle. Surround yourself with positive and like-minded individuals who uplift and inspire you. Nurture your relationships through open communication, active listening, empathy, and kindness. Practice forgiveness, compassion, and gratitude, fostering harmonious connections that contribute to your overall well-being.

Connecting with Nature:

Spending time in nature is deeply nourishing for the body, mind, and spirit. Take walks in natural surroundings, practice grounding techniques like barefoot walking, or simply sit and observe the beauty of the natural world. Connecting with nature promotes a sense of interconnectedness, calmness, and harmony, helping to reduce stress and rejuvenate your energy.

Cultivating a Positive Environment:

Create a positive and serene environment in your living space. Declutter, organize, and create a clean and harmonious home environment. Surround yourself with uplifting and inspiring elements such as plants, natural light, soothing colors, and meaningful artwork. Minimize exposure to negative influences like excessive noise, artificial lighting, and electronic devices, especially during restful times.

Practicing Gratitude and Service:

Expressing gratitude for the blessings in your life is a powerful practice that shifts your focus to positivity and abundance. Take time each day to acknowledge and appreciate the simple joys and experiences. Engaging in acts of service and kindness towards others promotes a sense of purpose, connection, and fulfillment. Offering selfless service uplifts not only others but also your own well-being.

By incorporating these Sattvic lifestyle practices into your daily routine, you can cultivate a balanced and harmonious way of living. Embracing these practices supports holistic wellness, promotes self-awareness, and nurtures the integration of body, mind, and spirit. Remember that these practices are a journey, and the key is consistency and finding what resonates with you on your path to well-being.

5.1 DAILY ROUTINE AND SELF-CARE RITUALS

A well-designed daily routine and self-care rituals are essential components of a Sattvic lifestyle. They provide structure, balance, and nourishment for the body, mind, and spirit. By incorporating intentional practices into your daily routine, you can cultivate a sense of well-being, inner harmony, and optimal health. Let's explore some key elements of a Sattvic daily routine and self-care rituals:

Wake Up Early:

In the Sattvic tradition, waking up early, ideally before sunrise, is encouraged. This time of the day, known as "Brahma muhurta," is considered auspicious and conducive to clarity, peace, and spiritual practice. Rising early allows you to start the day with a sense of calmness and gives you time for self-care practices.

Cleansing Practices:

Upon waking, engage in cleansing practices to refresh and awaken the body. These may include:

Tongue scraping: Use a tongue scraper or the back of a spoon to gently scrape your tongue, removing any toxins or residue accumulated overnight.

Oil pulling: Swish a tablespoon of organic sesame or coconut oil in your mouth for a few minutes, then spit it out. Oil pulling helps remove toxins and promotes oral health.

Warm water with lemon: Squeeze fresh lemon juice into a glass of warm water and drink it. This helps alkalize the body, supports digestion, and hydrates the system.

Meditation and Mindfulness:

Start your day with a period of meditation or mindfulness practice. Find a quiet and comfortable space where you can sit in stillness and connect with your inner self. Choose a meditation technique that resonates with you, such as focusing on the breath, repeating a mantra, or practicing mindfulness. This practice cultivates mental clarity, reduces stress, and sets a positive tone for the day ahead.

Movement and Exercise:

Engage in gentle movement or exercise to invigorate the body and promote circulation. This can include practices like yoga, stretching, walking, or any form of exercise that suits your preferences and needs. Aim for at least 30 minutes of physical activity each day to support overall health, flexibility, and vitality.

Sattvic Breakfast:

Enjoy a nourishing and Sattvic breakfast to provide essential nutrients and energy for the day. Choose foods that are light, fresh, and easy to digest, such as fresh fruits, cooked grains like quinoa or millet, herbal teas, and natural sweeteners like honey or jaggery. Avoid heavy or processed foods that may weigh you down or disturb your digestion.

Work and Productivity:

Structure your work or daily activities in a way that allows for focused and productive periods, balanced with regular breaks. Prioritize tasks based on importance and urgency, and practice time management techniques to optimize productivity. Take short breaks to rest, stretch, or engage in mindfulness practices throughout the day.

Mindful Eating:

Approach your meals with mindfulness and awareness. Sit down in a calm environment, free from distractions, and savor each bite of your food. Chew slowly and thoroughly, allowing your body to fully process and absorb the nutrients. Cultivate gratitude for the nourishment provided by the food and listen to your body's cues of hunger and fullness.

Self-Care Rituals:

Incorporate self-care rituals into your daily routine to nurture your body, mind, and spirit. These may include:

Gentle self-massage: Use warm oil, such as sesame or coconut oil, to massage your body, promoting relaxation, circulation, and skin health.

Bathing or showering: Take a refreshing bath or shower to cleanse and rejuvenate your body. Consider adding natural essential oils or bath salts for an added sensory experience.

Daily affirmations: Practice positive affirmations or self-empowering statements to cultivate a positive mindset and nurture self-belief.

Gratitude journaling: Take a few moments each day to write down things you are grateful for. This practice promotes a sense of appreciation and shifts your focus towards positivity.

Rest and relaxation: Set aside time for rest and relaxation, whether it's through meditation, reading, listening to soothing music, or engaging in hobbies that bring you joy.

Evening Wind-Down:

Create a calming evening routine to signal to your body and mind that it's time to unwind and prepare for restful sleep. Dim the lights, disconnect from electronic devices, and engage in activities that promote relaxation, such as gentle stretching, reading a book, practicing deep breathing exercises, or enjoying a cup of herbal tea.

Adequate Sleep:

Prioritize quality sleep by establishing a consistent sleep schedule and creating a peaceful sleep environment. Aim for 7-8 hours of uninterrupted sleep each night to allow your body to rest, repair, and rejuvenate.

Remember, a daily routine and self-care rituals are personal and can be tailored to suit your preferences and lifestyle. The key is to create a routine that supports balance, nourishment, and self-awareness. Experiment with different practices and listen to your body's needs to find what works best for you. With time and consistency, a Sattvic daily routine will become a foundation for holistic well-being and a source of inner harmony.

5.2 YOGA ASANAS FOR BALANCING BODY AND MIND

Yoga is an ancient practice that encompasses physical postures, breath control, and meditation to promote harmony and balance in the body and mind. The practice of yoga asanas, or postures, is a powerful tool for cultivating strength, flexibility, and inner calm. Through a combination of mindful movement and focused breathing, yoga helps release physical tension, increase energy flow, and bring a sense of balance and harmony to the body-mind complex. Let's explore some key yoga asanas for balancing the body and mind:

Mountain Pose (Tadasana):

This foundational pose establishes a strong and grounded foundation. Stand with your feet hip-width apart, aligning your body from the crown of your head to the soles of your feet. Engage your core, relax your shoulders, and breathe deeply. Mountain Pose helps improve posture, enhances body awareness, and promotes a sense of stability and groundedness.

Tree Pose (Vrikshasana):

Tree Pose helps improve balance and focus. Stand tall and shift your weight onto one leg, placing the sole of the opposite foot on the inner thigh or calf of the standing leg. Keep your gaze steady and bring your hands to your heart center or extend them overhead. Tree Pose strengthens the legs, improves concentration, and cultivates a sense of rootedness and balance.

Warrior Pose (Virabhadrasana):

Warrior Pose builds strength, stability, and confidence. Step your feet wide apart, turn one foot out, and bend the front knee, keeping the back leg straight. Raise your arms parallel to the floor, with your gaze focused forward. Warrior Pose strengthens the legs, opens the chest and shoulders, and fosters a sense of empowerment and determination.

Child's Pose (Balasana):

Child's Pose is a restorative pose that promotes relaxation and release. Kneel on the floor, bring your big toes together, and sit back on your heels. Lower your torso between your thighs and rest your forehead on the floor. Extend your arms forward or alongside your body. Child's Pose gently stretches the lower back, hips, and shoulders, allowing for deep relaxation and a sense of surrender.

Cat-Cow Pose (Marjaryasana-Bitilasana):

Cat-Cow Pose is a gentle flowing movement that helps release tension in the spine and promote flexibility. Start on your hands and knees, aligning your wrists under your shoulders and your knees under your hips. On the inhale, arch your back and lift your tailbone, allowing your belly to sink towards the floor (Cow Pose). On the exhale, round your spine, tuck your tailbone, and draw your belly button towards your spine (Cat Pose). Cat-Cow Pose stretches the spine, massages the organs, and enhances spinal flexibility.

Downward-Facing Dog (Adho Mukha Svanasana):

Downward-Facing Dog is a rejuvenating pose that stretches the entire body. Start on your hands and knees, tuck your toes, and lift your hips up towards the ceiling, forming an inverted V shape. Keep your hands shoulder-width apart and your feet hip-width apart. Press your hands into the mat, lengthen your spine, and relax your heels towards the floor. Downward-Facing Dog lengthens the spine, stretches the hamstrings, and rejuvenates the body and mind.

Corpse Pose (Savasana):

Corpse Pose is a relaxation pose that allows the body to integrate the benefits of the practice. Lie flat on your back, arms extended alongside your body, palms facing up. Close your eyes and consciously relax every part of your body, from your toes to the top of your head. Focus on your breath and allow your mind to enter a state of deep relaxation. Corpse Pose rejuvenates the body, calms the nervous system, and promotes a sense of deep rest and integration.

Remember to approach yoga asanas with awareness, respect your body's limits, and honor your individual needs. It's always beneficial to practice under the guidance of a qualified yoga teacher, especially if you're new to yoga or have specific health concerns. Regular practice of these yoga asanas can help create a balanced and harmonious state within the body and mind, fostering overall well-being and inner peace.

5.3 PRANAYAMA TECHNIQUES FOR VITAL ENERGY FLOW

Pranayama, the practice of breath control, is an integral aspect of yoga and the Sattvic lifestyle. It involves conscious regulation of the breath to enhance the flow of vital energy (prana) in the body, promoting physical and mental well-being. Pranayama techniques offer numerous benefits, including stress reduction, increased focus, improved respiratory function, and heightened self-awareness. Let's explore some key pranayama techniques for vital energy flow:

Dirga Pranayama (Three-Part Breath):

Dirga Pranayama is a foundational breathing technique that promotes deep relaxation and stress relief. Start by sitting in a comfortable position. Inhale deeply through your nose, filling your abdomen, then your rib cage, and finally your chest. Exhale slowly, releasing the breath from your chest, rib cage, and abdomen. Repeat this three-part breath, focusing on smooth and even inhalations and exhalations. Dirga Pranayama nourishes the body with oxygen, calms the mind, and supports overall well-being.

Nadi Shodhana (Alternate Nostril Breathing):

Nadi Shodhana is a balancing and purifying pranayama technique that harmonizes the flow of energy in the body. Sit comfortably and use your right hand to close your right nostril with your thumb. Inhale deeply through your left nostril, then close it with your ring finger. Release the right nostril and exhale through it. Inhale through the right nostril, close it, and exhale through the left. Continue alternating the breath, focusing on smooth and steady inhalations and exhalations. Nadi Shodhana balances the left and right energy channels, calms the mind, and promotes mental clarity.

Ujjayi Pranayama (Victorious Breath):

Ujjayi Pranayama is a deep, audible breath that cultivates internal heat and focus. Sit comfortably and slightly constrict the back of your throat, creating a soft hissing sound as you breathe in and out through your nose. Take slow, deep breaths, ensuring that the inhalations and exhalations are equal in length. Ujjayi Pranayama helps increase oxygenation, regulates body temperature, and enhances concentration.

Kapalabhati (Skull Shining Breath):

Kapalabhati is an energizing and cleansing pranayama technique that involves rapid exhalations and passive inhalations. Sit with your spine straight and take a deep breath in. Exhale forcefully by quickly contracting your abdominal muscles, pushing the breath out through your nose. The inhalation happens naturally as you relax your abdomen. Start with a few rounds of slow-paced Kapalabhati and gradually increase the speed. Kapalabhati stimulates the abdominal organs, releases toxins, and invigorates the body and mind.

Sheetali Pranayama (Cooling Breath):

Sheetali Pranayama is a cooling breath technique that helps reduce body heat and soothe the nervous system. Roll your tongue into a tube shape or slightly part your lips if you can't roll your tongue. Inhale slowly through the rolled tongue or parted lips, drawing the breath in a cooling manner. Close your mouth and exhale gently through your nose. Continue for several rounds. Sheetali Pranayama calms the mind, reduces stress, and cools the body's internal temperature.

Bhramari Pranayama (Bee Breath):

Bhramari Pranayama is a calming and meditative breathing technique that mimics the soothing sound of a buzzing bee. Sit comfortably and close your eyes. Place your index fingers on your ears, gently pressing the cartilage to close them partially. Inhale deeply through your nose, and as you exhale, make a humming sound like a bee, allowing the sound to resonate in your head. Repeat for several rounds. Bhramari Pranayama calms the mind, relieves anxiety, and promotes a sense of inner peace.

When practicing pranayama, it's essential to start slowly, pay attention to the sensations in your body, and never force the breath. If you have any respiratory conditions or health concerns, consult with a qualified yoga teacher or healthcare professional before engaging in pranayama practices. Regular practice of these pranayama techniques can help enhance the flow of vital energy, balance the body-mind complex, and promote overall vitality and well-being.

5.4 CREATING A SERENE SATTVIC ENVIRONMENT

The environment we surround ourselves with has a significant impact on our well-being, energy levels, and overall state of mind. In the context of the Sattvic lifestyle, creating a serene environment becomes crucial in supporting our journey towards inner harmony and balance. A serene Sattvic environment encompasses elements that promote calmness, purity, and positive energy. Here are some key considerations for creating a serene Sattvic environment:

Declutter and Simplify:

Start by decluttering your physical space. Remove unnecessary items and organize your belongings in a way that promotes a sense of order and simplicity. Clutter can create mental and emotional unrest, while a tidy environment helps clear the mind and create a peaceful atmosphere.

Natural Elements:

Incorporate natural elements into your space to connect with the healing power of nature. Bring in plants, flowers, and natural materials such as wood, stone, or cotton. These elements not only beautify the space but also contribute to a sense of harmony and connection with the natural world.

Harmonious Colors:

Choose colors that evoke a sense of calmness and serenity. Soft pastel shades, earthy tones, and shades of white can create a soothing and serene atmosphere. Avoid overly bright or stimulating colors, as they may disrupt the peaceful ambiance.

Lighting:

Pay attention to lighting in your environment. Natural light is ideal, so keep curtains and blinds open during the day to let sunlight in. Use soft and warm artificial lighting in the evenings to create a cozy and tranquil ambiance. Avoid harsh or fluorescent lighting, as it can create a sense of tension and restlessness.

Mindful Arrangement:

Arrange furniture and objects in a way that promotes flow and harmony. Create open spaces and avoid cluttered arrangements that hinder movement and energy flow. Consider the principles of Feng Shui or Vastu Shastra, ancient systems of spatial arrangement, to optimize the energy flow within your space.

Sacred Symbols and Inspirational Art:

Decorate your space with sacred symbols, meaningful artwork, and inspirational quotes or affirmations. These elements can serve as reminders of your spiritual journey and aspirations, fostering a positive and uplifting environment.

Aromatherapy:

Engage your sense of smell by using essential oils or incense that promote relaxation and a sense of well-being. Lavender, sandalwood, rose, and citrus oils are known for their calming and uplifting properties. Use a diffuser or simply sprinkle a few drops onto a cloth or tissue to infuse the space with soothing scents.

Tranquil Sounds:

Create a serene auditory environment by playing soft instrumental music, nature sounds, or chants. These gentle sounds can help mask external noise, promote relaxation, and create a tranquil atmosphere.

Sacred Space for Meditation and Reflection:

Designate a specific area in your home as a sacred space for meditation, reflection, and spiritual practices. This can be a corner of a room or a dedicated room, adorned with cushions, candles, sacred objects, and anything that inspires and supports your inner journey.

Digital Detox:

Limit the presence of electronic devices and the distractions they bring. Set boundaries for screen time and create device-free zones in your home, especially in areas designated for relaxation and rejuvenation.

Remember, creating a serene Sattvic environment is a continuous process that requires mindfulness and conscious effort. Regularly reassess your space and make adjustments as needed to align with your evolving needs and spiritual journey. By cultivating a serene environment, you create a nurturing space that supports your physical, mental, and spiritual well-being, fostering a deep sense of inner peace and harmony.

6.THE SATTVIC DIET FOR DIFFERENT LIFE STAGES

The Sattvic diet is a holistic approach to nutrition that aims to promote balance and harmony in the body, mind, and spirit. It emphasizes the consumption of fresh, plant-based foods that are considered pure, nourishing, and light. While the basic principles of the Sattvic diet remain the same across different life stages, certain considerations can be made to meet the specific nutritional needs of individuals at different ages and life stages. Let's explore how the Sattvic diet can be adapted for various life stages:

Infants and Toddlers:

During the early stages of life, breast milk is the ideal source of nutrition for infants. Breast milk provides all the necessary nutrients and immune factors needed for healthy growth and development. If breastfeeding is not possible, consult with a healthcare professional to choose an appropriate formula. As toddlers transition to solid foods, introduce Sattvic foods gradually. Offer a variety of cooked and mashed fruits, vegetables, lentils, and grains in their diet. Avoid processed and refined foods, excessive spices, and sugary snacks.

Children and Adolescents:

Children and adolescents have higher energy and nutrient

requirements due to their rapid growth and development. The Sattvic diet can provide them with essential nutrients while nurturing their overall well-being. Emphasize a variety of whole grains, fruits, vegetables, legumes, nuts, and seeds in their meals. Include dairy products like milk, yogurt, and ghee, if they are well-tolerated. Offer healthy snacks like fresh fruits, homemade energy bars, and nuts. Limit their intake of processed and sugary foods, and encourage them to drink plenty of water.

Adults:

For adults, the Sattvic diet offers a balanced and nourishing approach to nutrition. Emphasize a variety of fresh, seasonal fruits and vegetables, whole grains, legumes, nuts, seeds, and dairy products (if well-tolerated). Include a moderate amount of plant-based proteins like tofu, tempeh, and seitan. Opt for cooking methods that retain the natural flavors and nutrients of the ingredients, such as steaming, boiling, sautéing, and baking. Use natural sweeteners like honey or jaggery instead of refined sugar. Stay hydrated by drinking sufficient water and herbal teas. It is also important to listen to your body's needs and adjust portion sizes accordingly.

Pregnant and Nursing Women:

Pregnancy and lactation require additional nutrients to support the growth and development of the baby. During pregnancy, focus on consuming nutrient-dense foods such as leafy greens, colorful vegetables, whole grains, legumes, and seeds. Ensure an adequate intake of calcium, iron, folate, and omega-3 fatty acids. Include sources of plant-based proteins and healthy fats. Consult with a healthcare professional for personalized guidance on supplementation, if necessary. Nursing women should continue to follow a balanced Sattvic diet and drink plenty of fluids to support milk production.

Elderly Individuals:

As we age, our nutritional needs may change, and certain health conditions may arise. The Sattvic diet can be tailored to accommodate the specific needs of elderly individuals. Emphasize easily digestible foods, such as cooked vegetables, whole grains, soups, and stews. Include sources of lean proteins, such as legumes, tofu, and dairy products (if well-tolerated). Adequate intake of fiber, vitamins, and minerals is essential for maintaining optimal health. Consider consulting with a healthcare professional or a registered dietitian for personalized guidance based on individual health conditions and medications.

It's important to note that the information provided here is general in nature, and individual nutritional needs may vary. If you have specific dietary concerns or health conditions, it's advisable to consult with a qualified healthcare professional or a registered dietitian for personalized guidance on incorporating the Sattvic diet into different life stages.

6.1 SATTVIC NUTRITION FOR CHILDREN AND TEENS

Proper nutrition is crucial for the growth, development, and overall well-being of children and teens. The Sattvic diet offers a balanced and nourishing approach to nutrition that can support their physical, mental, and emotional health. Here's an extensive guide to Sattvic nutrition for children and teens:

Emphasize Whole Foods:

The Sattvic diet places a strong emphasis on whole, unprocessed foods. Encourage children and teens to consume a variety of fresh fruits, vegetables, whole grains, legumes, nuts, and seeds. These foods are rich in essential nutrients, fiber, and antioxidants, supporting their overall growth and development.

Opt for Organic and Seasonal Foods:

Whenever possible, choose organic and locally grown foods. Organic produce is free from harmful pesticides and chemicals, promoting a healthier and cleaner diet. Additionally, opt for seasonal foods as they tend to be fresher and more nutrient-dense.

Balanced Macronutrients:

Ensure a balance of macronutrients in their meals. Include adequate sources of carbohydrates (whole grains, fruits, and vegetables), proteins (legumes, nuts, seeds, and dairy products if well-tolerated), and healthy fats (avocado, nuts, seeds, and cold-pressed oils). This balance helps provide sustained energy, support growth, and maintain overall health.

Adequate Protein Intake:

Protein is essential for children and teens as they undergo rapid growth and development. Include plant-based protein sources such as lentils, chickpeas, tofu, tempeh, and quinoa. If they consume dairy, include yogurt, cottage cheese, or paneer as additional sources of protein.

Calcium-Rich Foods:

Calcium is vital for developing strong bones and teeth. Incorporate calcium-rich foods such as milk (if well-tolerated), yogurt, cheese, almonds, sesame seeds, and leafy green vegetables like spinach and kale. If needed, consult a healthcare professional or registered dietitian for guidance on calcium supplementation.

Healthy Snacks:

Encourage healthy snacking options. Offer fresh fruits, homemade energy bars, raw nuts, and seeds as nutritious alternatives to processed snacks. Limit their intake of sugary treats, refined grains, and packaged snacks high in unhealthy fats.

Hydration:

Ensure children and teens drink sufficient water throughout the day to stay hydrated. Encourage them to carry a water bottle and develop the habit of drinking water regularly. Avoid excessive consumption of sugary beverages and opt for fresh fruit juices or herbal teas instead.

Mindful Eating:

Teach children and teens the importance of mindful eating. Encourage them to eat slowly, savor their food, and pay attention to hunger and fullness cues. Discourage distractions such as screens during mealtime to promote a mindful and enjoyable dining experience.

Cooking and Food Preparation:

Involve children and teens in meal planning, grocery shopping, and food preparation. This helps them develop a connection with food, appreciate the importance of nutrition, and learn valuable culinary skills.

Individual Needs and Preferences:

Respect individual needs and preferences when it comes to food choices. Some children may have specific dietary requirements or restrictions. Accommodate their needs while ensuring they still receive a balanced and nourishing diet. Consult with a healthcare professional or registered dietitian if you have specific concerns or questions.

Balanced Approach:

While the Sattvic diet provides a foundation for healthy eating, it's important to adopt a balanced approach. Allow for occasional treats and special indulgences to avoid creating a restrictive relationship with food. Teach children and teens about the importance of moderation and making informed food choices.

Role Modeling:

As parents and caregivers, be role models for healthy eating habits. Demonstrate the importance of consuming a balanced Sattvic diet by incorporating these principles into your own meals. Children are more likely to adopt healthy habits when they see their loved ones practicing them.

Remember, each child is unique, and their nutritional needs may vary. It's recommended to consult with a healthcare professional or registered dietitian to ensure individualized guidance based on specific requirements, growth stages, and any existing health conditions.

6.2 SATTVIC DIET DURING PREGNANCY AND POSTPARTUM

The Sattvic diet offers a holistic and nourishing approach to nutrition, making it particularly beneficial during the transformative phases of pregnancy and postpartum. By following the principles of the Sattvic diet, expectant mothers can provide optimal nutrition for themselves and their growing baby, while supporting their overall well-being. Here's an extensive guide to the Sattvic diet during pregnancy and postpartum:

During Pregnancy:

Balanced Nutrition: Focus on consuming a well-balanced diet that includes a variety of fresh fruits, vegetables, whole grains, legumes, nuts, seeds, and dairy products (if well-tolerated). Aim to meet increased nutritional requirements for pregnancy, including additional protein, iron, calcium, folate, and omega-3 fatty acids.

Plant-Based Proteins: Include plant-based protein sources such as lentils, chickpeas, quinoa, tofu, tempeh, and nuts. These provide essential amino acids for fetal growth and development.

Iron-Rich Foods: Incorporate iron-rich foods such as leafy green vegetables, dried fruits, legumes, and fortified whole grains. Pair them with a source of vitamin C, like citrus fruits, to enhance iron absorption.

Calcium Sources: Ensure an adequate intake of calcium for the development of the baby's bones and teeth. Include dairy products (if well-tolerated), yogurt, cheese, almonds, sesame seeds, and leafy green vegetables in your diet. Consult with a healthcare professional or registered dietitian for guidance on calcium supplementation, if needed.

Essential Fatty Acids: Include sources of omega-3 fatty acids, such as chia seeds, flaxseeds, walnuts, and cold-water fish (if consumed). These are important for the baby's brain and eye development.

Hydration: Drink plenty of water throughout the day to stay hydrated and support healthy blood circulation and amniotic fluid levels. Avoid excessive caffeine and opt for herbal teas or infused water instead.

Mindful Eating: Practice mindful eating by paying attention to hunger and fullness cues. Eat small, frequent meals to prevent discomfort from overeating or indigestion. Choose whole, unprocessed foods whenever possible.

Healthy Snacks: Opt for nourishing snacks like fresh fruits, yogurt, nuts, seeds, and homemade energy bars. Avoid processed and sugary snacks that provide empty calories.

Food Safety: Take precautions to ensure food safety during pregnancy. Avoid raw or undercooked seafood, meat, and eggs. Wash fruits and vegetables thoroughly, and practice good hygiene when handling food.

During Postpartum:

Adequate Nutrition: The postpartum period is a time of recovery and adjustment. Continue to prioritize a balanced and nourishing diet that supports healing and provides the necessary energy for breastfeeding and caring for your newborn.

Nutrient-Dense Foods: Include nutrient-dense foods such as fresh fruits, vegetables, whole grains, lean proteins, and healthy fats in your meals. These foods provide essential nutrients and support lactation.

Hydration: Stay hydrated by drinking sufficient water throughout the day, as breastfeeding increases fluid needs. Include herbal teas and soups to promote hydration and nourishment.

Caloric Needs: Ensure an adequate intake of calories to meet the increased energy demands of breastfeeding. Consult with a healthcare professional or registered dietitian to determine your individual calorie needs.

Galactagogues: Incorporate galactagogue foods into your diet to support milk production. These include fenugreek seeds, fennel seeds, cumin seeds, oats, and almonds. Consult with a healthcare professional for guidance on galactagogue supplementation if needed.

Postpartum Healing Foods: Include foods that support postpartum healing, such as turmeric, ginger, garlic, and spices like cumin and coriander. These foods have anti-inflammatory properties and can aid in wound healing.

Self-Care: Prioritize self-care and rest during the postpartum period. Focus on nourishing your body with healthy meals, practicing relaxation techniques, and seeking support from loved ones.

6.3 SATTVIC NUTRITION FOR AGING AND LONGEVITY

The Sattvic diet offers valuable principles that can support healthy aging and promote longevity. By adopting a Sattvic approach to nutrition, individuals can provide their bodies with nourishing foods that support vitality, mental clarity, and overall well-being as they age. Here's an extensive guide to Sattvic nutrition for aging and longevity:

Nutrient-Dense Foods: Emphasize nutrient-dense foods that provide a wide range of vitamins, minerals, antioxidants, and phytochemicals. Include a variety of fresh fruits, vegetables, whole grains, legumes, nuts, seeds, and dairy products (if well-tolerated). These foods provide essential nutrients necessary for optimal bodily function and support overall health.

Antioxidant-Rich Foods: Include foods that are rich in antioxidants, such as berries, dark leafy greens, cruciferous vegetables, turmeric, green tea, and cacao. Antioxidants help protect the body against oxidative stress and cellular damage, promoting healthy aging.

Omega-3 Fatty Acids: Incorporate sources of omega-3 fatty acids into your diet, such as fatty fish (e.g., salmon, sardines), flaxseeds, chia seeds, and walnuts. Omega-3 fatty acids support brain health, reduce inflammation, and promote cardiovascular health.

Adequate Protein Intake: Ensure a sufficient intake of high-quality protein to support muscle health and maintenance. Include lean sources of protein such as legumes, tofu, tempeh, nuts, seeds, and if well-tolerated, dairy products. Protein also supports immune function, tissue repair, and hormone production.

Fiber-Rich Foods: Consume an ample amount of dietary fiber through fruits, vegetables, whole grains, and legumes. Fiber aids in digestion, supports gut health, helps manage weight, and reduces the risk of chronic diseases such as cardiovascular disease and type 2 diabetes.

Hydration: Stay hydrated by drinking plenty of water throughout the day. Sufficient hydration is important for maintaining proper bodily functions, promoting healthy skin, and supporting cognitive function.

Mindful Eating: Practice mindful eating by savoring each bite, chewing thoroughly, and paying attention to hunger and satiety cues. Slow down during meals, and cultivate a relaxed and peaceful eating environment.

Herbal Teas and Infusions: Incorporate herbal teas and infusions into your daily routine. Opt for calming and rejuvenating herbs such as chamomile, holy basil (tulsi), peppermint, and rosemary. These herbs can have soothing effects on the body and support overall well-being.

Moderation and Balance: Practice moderation and balance in your dietary choices. Avoid excessive intake of processed foods, refined sugars, unhealthy fats, and sodium. Instead, focus on whole, unprocessed foods and prepare meals at home whenever possible.

Regular Physical Activity: Combine a Sattvic diet with regular physical activity to promote longevity and overall health. Engage in activities that you enjoy, such as walking, yoga, swimming, or strength training. Regular exercise can improve cardiovascular health, maintain muscle mass, enhance mood, and support overall well-being.

Social Connection: Foster social connections and engage in meaningful relationships. Strong social ties are associated with better mental health, emotional well-being, and cognitive function, contributing to a higher quality of life as you age.

Mind-Body Practices: Explore mind-body practices such as meditation, yoga, tai chi, or qigong. These practices can help reduce stress, promote mental clarity, and enhance overall resilience and well-being.

Individual nutritional needs may vary, and it's important to consider any specific health conditions, medications, or dietary restrictions when implementing dietary changes. It's advisable to consult with a healthcare professional or registered dietitian for personalized guidance and support tailored to your needs and goals for healthy aging and longevity.

7.INTEGRATING THE SATTVIC DIET INTO MODERN LIFE

The Sattvic diet, with its emphasis on fresh, whole, and balanced foods, can be integrated into modern lifestyles to promote health, well-being, and harmony. While modern life often comes with its own set of challenges, incorporating Sattvic principles into your daily routine can help you navigate the demands of contemporary living while nurturing your body, mind, and spirit. Here's an extensive guide on integrating the Sattvic diet into modern life:

Meal Planning and Preparation:

Set aside time for meal planning and grocery shopping to ensure you have a variety of Sattvic ingredients on hand.

Batch cook and meal prep to save time during busy weekdays.

Experiment with Sattvic recipes and adapt them to your taste preferences.

Mindful Eating:

Practice mindful eating by slowing down, savoring each bite, and paying attention to your body's hunger and fullness signals.

Create a calm and peaceful eating environment, free from distractions like screens or stressful conversations.

Chew your food thoroughly and appreciate the flavors, textures, and aromas of the Sattvic ingredients.

Sattvic Snacking:

Keep healthy Sattvic snacks readily available, such as fresh fruits, nuts, seeds, homemade energy balls, or vegetable sticks with hummus.

Avoid processed and unhealthy snacks, opting for nourishing options that support your well-being throughout the day.

Conscious Food Choices:

Make conscious choices when it comes to food sourcing. Select organic, locally grown, and seasonal produce whenever possible to support sustainability and minimize exposure to pesticides and chemicals.

Choose whole, unprocessed foods over packaged and processed options, which often contain additives, preservatives, and excessive amounts of salt, sugar, and unhealthy fats.

Eating Out Mindfully:

When dining out, choose restaurants that offer Sattvic-inspired dishes or those that prioritize fresh, whole ingredients.

Be mindful of portion sizes and avoid overeating. Listen to your body's cues of satiety.

Request modifications to dishes, such as replacing unhealthy cooking oils with healthier alternatives like ghee or olive oil.

Socializing and Sharing Sattvic Meals:

Invite friends and family to share Sattvic meals together. Explain the principles and benefits of the Sattvic diet to encourage their participation and understanding.

Explore potluck gatherings where everyone contributes a Sattvic-inspired dish, creating a diverse and nourishing meal.

Food Mindfulness in the Workplace:

Pack your own Sattvic-inspired lunches for work to ensure you have control over the ingredients and nutritional quality of your meals.

Find Sattvic options in nearby cafeterias or restaurants if eating out during work hours.

Take short breaks to eat mindfully, away from your desk, and focus on nourishing your body and mind.

Balancing Technology and Sattvic Lifestyle:

Set boundaries with technology to create space for mindful eating, self-reflection, and connection with nature.

Use technology to your advantage by exploring Sattvic recipes, educational resources, and meditation apps that support your Sattvic lifestyle.

Sattvic Lifestyle Practices:

Beyond diet, incorporate other Sattvic lifestyle practices, such as yoga, meditation, pranayama (breathing exercises), and self-care rituals, into your daily routine.

Prioritize restful sleep, regular physical activity, and meaningful social connections to support overall well-being.

Personalize and Adapt:

Remember that the Sattvic diet is a flexible framework. Personalize it to suit your individual needs, tastes, and cultural preferences while staying true to the principles of balance, freshness, and wholesomeness.

By integrating the Sattvic diet into modern life, you can cultivate a sense of harmony, nourish your body, and enhance your overall well-being. Experiment with different Sattvic recipes, be open to new flavors and ingredients, and embrace the journey of exploring this ancient and holistic approach to nutrition.

7.1 OVERCOMING CHALLENGES AND ADAPTING TO CONTEMPORARY LIFESTYLES

Incorporating the Sattvic diet into a contemporary lifestyle may present certain challenges, but with awareness, planning, and adaptation, it is possible to overcome these obstacles and reap the benefits of this wholesome and balanced approach to nutrition. Here's an extensive guide on overcoming challenges and adapting the Sattvic diet to fit modern lifestyles:

Time Constraints:

Plan and prepare meals in advance: Set aside dedicated time for meal planning, grocery shopping, and food preparation to ensure you have Sattvic ingredients readily available.

Batch cooking: Cook larger quantities of Sattvic dishes and store them in the refrigerator or freezer for convenient and quick meals during busy days.

Simplify recipes: Choose recipes that require minimal preparation and cooking time. Focus on simple, nourishing meals that can be prepared in a short amount of time.

Availability of Ingredients:

Explore local markets and health food stores: Look for stores that specialize in organic produce and whole foods. These establishments often carry a wide variety of Sattvic ingredients.

Online shopping: Utilize online platforms to access a broader range of Sattvic ingredients that may not be readily available in your local area.

Seasonal eating: Embrace the concept of eating seasonally and prioritize fresh, local produce. Adjust your meal plans according to the availability of seasonal fruits and vegetables.

Social Situations and Dining Out:

Communicate your dietary preferences: Inform friends, family, and hosts about your Sattvic dietary choices. Explain the principles and benefits of the Sattvic diet, and offer to contribute a Sattvic dish to social gatherings.

Research restaurants: Before dining out, research restaurants that offer Sattvic-friendly options or those that prioritize fresh, whole ingredients. Check menus in advance and inquire about customization options.

Flexibility and moderation: While it's ideal to adhere to the Sattvic diet as closely as possible, be flexible in social situations. Make the best choices available, opting for healthier options and moderating your intake of non-Sattvic foods.

Travel and Eating On-the-Go:

Plan ahead: Pack Sattvic snacks, such as nuts, seeds, fresh fruits, or homemade energy bars, to have nutritious options readily available while traveling.

Research local cuisine: Prior to your trip, learn about the local cuisine and identify Sattvic dishes or ingredients that you can enjoy. This will help you make informed choices while dining out or exploring local markets.

Carry a water bottle: Stay hydrated by carrying a reusable water bottle and refilling it throughout the day.

Emotional and Craving-Based Eating:

Mindful awareness: Practice mindful eating and develop awareness of your emotional triggers and cravings. Pause before indulging in non-Sattvic foods and consider alternative ways to address emotional needs or cravings, such as engaging in a stress-relieving activity or enjoying a Sattvic snack.

Support and Accountability:

Find like-minded individuals: Seek out communities or support groups that share an interest in the Sattvic lifestyle. Connect with others who can provide encouragement, recipe ideas, and tips for overcoming challenges.

Enlist a buddy: Partner with a friend or family member who is also interested in the Sattvic diet. Share meal plans, cook together, and hold each other accountable for staying on track.

Flexibility and Adaptation:

Customize the diet to fit your needs: The Sattvic diet is a flexible framework. Tailor it to suit your individual dietary preferences, cultural background, and health requirements. Be open to modifications and adaptations that align with the core principles of balance, freshness, and wholesomeness.

The Sattvic diet is not about perfection but rather about making conscious choices and cultivating a balanced approach to nutrition. Embrace the journey of incorporating Sattvic principles into your contemporary lifestyle, and be patient with yourself as you navigate challenges and adapt to this nourishing way of eating

7.2 SATTVIC DIET FOR WEIGHT MANAGEMENT AND DETOXIFICATION

The Sattvic diet, with its emphasis on fresh, whole, and balanced foods, can be a valuable tool for weight management and detoxification. By adopting Sattvic principles in your dietary choices, you can support your body's natural detoxification processes, maintain a healthy weight, and promote overall well-being. Here's an extensive guide on using the Sattvic diet for weight management and detoxification:

1. Focus on Whole, Plant-Based Foods:
    - Prioritize whole grains like brown rice, quinoa, and millet, as well as legumes such as lentils, chickpeas, and mung beans. These provide essential nutrients, fiber, and sustained energy.

    - Include a variety of fresh fruits and vegetables, both raw and cooked, to provide essential vitamins, minerals, and antioxidants.

    - Incorporate nuts, seeds, and healthy fats like avocado and coconut oil for satiety and to support cellular health.

2. Balance Macronutrients:
    - Aim for a balance of carbohydrates, proteins,

and healthy fats in your meals to promote stable blood sugar levels, sustained energy, and feelings of fullness.

- Opt for complex carbohydrates like whole grains, fruits, and vegetables, which provide sustained energy and promote feelings of satiety.

- Include lean sources of protein such as legumes, tofu, tempeh, and dairy products if included in your diet.

- Incorporate healthy fats from sources like nuts, seeds, avocados, and cold-pressed oils to support brain health, hormone balance, and nutrient absorption.

3. Portion Control:
   - Be mindful of portion sizes to avoid overeating and promote weight management.

   - Listen to your body's hunger and fullness cues. Eat until you feel satisfied, but not overly stuffed.

   - Consider using smaller plates and bowls to help control portion sizes and create a visual perception of a full meal.

4. Hydration:
   - Drink plenty of water throughout the day to support the body's detoxification processes and maintain optimal hydration.

   - Consider incorporating herbal teas or infused water with lemon, cucumber, or mint for added flavor and detoxifying benefits.

5. Limit Processed and Refined Foods:
   - Minimize or avoid processed and refined foods that are high in added sugars, unhealthy

fats, and artificial additives. These can hinder weight management efforts and contribute to toxin buildup in the body.

- Read food labels carefully and choose foods with minimal ingredients, focusing on whole, unprocessed options.

6. Emphasize Detoxifying Foods:
    - Include foods known for their detoxifying properties, such as bitter greens like kale, spinach, and dandelion greens. These help support liver function and aid in eliminating toxins from the body.

    - Include sulfur-rich foods like cruciferous vegetables (broccoli, cauliflower, cabbage) and onions, which assist in liver detoxification.

    - Incorporate foods rich in antioxidants, such as berries, turmeric, and green tea, to help combat oxidative stress and support overall detoxification.

7. Mindful Eating and Digestion:
    - Practice mindful eating by slowing down, chewing your food thoroughly, and savoring each bite. This promotes better digestion and allows your body to absorb nutrients more effectively.

    - Avoid distractions while eating, such as screens or stressful conversations, as they can interfere with proper digestion.

8. Regular Physical Activity:
    - Pair your Sattvic diet with regular physical activity to support weight management, strengthen your body, and enhance overall well-being.

- Engage in activities you enjoy, such as yoga, brisk walking, swimming, or cycling, to make exercise a sustainable part of your lifestyle.

9. Seek Professional Guidance:
    - If you have specific weight management goals or health concerns, it's advisable to consult a qualified healthcare professional or registered dietitian who can provide personalized guidance and support.

7.3 SUPPORTING MENTAL HEALTH WITH SATTVIC PRINCIPLES

The Sattvic diet and lifestyle, with their focus on balance, purity, and harmony, can greatly contribute to supporting mental health and emotional well-being. By embracing Sattvic principles, you can create a nourishing environment for your mind, cultivate emotional balance, and enhance your overall mental well-being. Here's an extensive guide on supporting mental health with Sattvic principles:

1. Nutrient-Dense Foods:
    - The Sattvic diet emphasizes whole, unprocessed, and nutrient-dense foods that provide essential vitamins, minerals, and antioxidants necessary for optimal brain function and mental well-being.
    - Include a variety of fruits and vegetables rich in antioxidants, such as berries, leafy greens, and colorful produce, which can help combat oxidative stress and support brain health.
    - Incorporate healthy fats from sources like nuts, seeds, avocados, and cold-pressed oils, as they provide essential omega-3 fatty acids that support brain health and help regulate mood.

2. Mind-Gut Connection:
    - The Sattvic diet promotes a healthy gut

microbiome, which plays a crucial role in mental health. Include probiotic-rich foods like yogurt, kefir, sauerkraut, and kimchi to support a healthy gut flora.

- Prioritize fiber-rich foods such as whole grains, legumes, and vegetables to promote healthy digestion and support the production of neurotransmitters that impact mood.

3. Balancing the Doshas:
   - According to Ayurveda, imbalances in the three doshas (Vata, Pitta, and Kapha) can contribute to mental health issues. The Sattvic diet aims to balance the doshas through its emphasis on fresh, whole foods and mindful eating practices.
   - Seek guidance from an Ayurvedic practitioner to understand your unique constitution and make dietary choices that support the balance of your doshas.

4. Mindful Eating Practices:
   - Practice mindful eating by paying attention to your food, savoring each bite, and eating in a calm and peaceful environment. This promotes better digestion and absorption of nutrients while fostering a deeper connection with your body's signals of hunger and fullness.
   - Avoid distractions while eating, such as screens or stressful conversations, and instead focus on the sensory experience of the food.

5. Limiting Stimulants:
   - Reduce or eliminate stimulants like caffeine, as they can exacerbate anxiety, disrupt sleep, and contribute to imbalances in the nervous system. Opt for caffeine-free herbal teas or

warm water with lemon for hydration and gentle relaxation.

6. Meditation and Mindfulness:
    - Regularly engage in meditation and mindfulness practices, which can help calm the mind, reduce stress, and cultivate inner peace.

    - Set aside dedicated time each day for meditation or mindfulness activities such as deep breathing exercises, guided visualizations, or gentle yoga practices.

7. Connecting with Nature:
    - Spend time in nature to support mental well-being. Engage in activities like walking, gardening, or simply sitting in a natural setting to foster a sense of peace and connection.

    - Incorporate seasonal and organic foods into your diet to align with the natural rhythms of the earth and promote a deeper connection with nature.

8. Emotional Balance and Self-Care:
    - Cultivate emotional balance by practicing self-care activities that nourish your mind and spirit. This can include activities like journaling, engaging in creative pursuits, spending time with loved ones, or engaging in relaxation techniques such as aromatherapy or gentle massages.

9. Seeking Support:
    - If you're experiencing persistent mental health challenges, it's important to seek professional support from a qualified mental health practitioner. They can provide guidance, therapies, and interventions tailored to your specific needs.

Mental health is a holistic aspect of well-being, and the Sattvic diet and lifestyle can be valuable tools in promoting mental well-being. By embracing Sattvic principles, nurturing your mind, and creating a harmonious lifestyle, you can support your mental health and enhance your overall sense of well-being.

8.SATTVIC DIET FOR SPIRITUAL GROWTH AND AWAKENING

The Sattvic diet, with its focus on purity, balance, and harmonious living, is deeply connected to spiritual growth and awakening. By adopting the Sattvic principles in your diet and lifestyle, you can create a conducive environment for spiritual development, enhance your connection to higher consciousness, and facilitate inner transformation. Here's an extensive guide on the Sattvic diet for spiritual growth and awakening:

1. Purification of Body and Mind:

   - The Sattvic diet aims to purify the body and mind, as they are considered vehicles for spiritual growth. By consuming fresh, natural, and minimally processed foods, you provide the body with the nourishment it needs while minimizing the intake of toxins and disturbances.

   - Avoid processed, artificially flavored, and chemically treated foods, as they can cloud the mind and create imbalance in the body.

2. Lightness and Prana:

   - Sattvic foods are believed to be light, easy to digest, and filled with life force energy or prana. These foods promote clarity of mind, increase vitality, and enhance the flow of energy throughout the body.

- Include fresh fruits, vegetables, whole grains, and plant-based proteins in your diet to maximize prana intake and support spiritual growth.

3. Mindful and Intentional Eating:

- Practice mindful and intentional eating to cultivate a deeper connection with your food and the nourishment it provides. Be fully present while eating, savoring each bite, and expressing gratitude for the sustenance it offers.

- Avoid distractions such as screens or stressful conversations while eating, and instead, create a calm and serene atmosphere that allows you to fully appreciate the flavors and textures of your food.

4. Non-violence (Ahimsa):

- Ahimsa, the principle of non-violence, is fundamental in the Sattvic diet. Choose foods that are obtained without harm to animals or the environment.

- Opt for plant-based protein sources such as legumes, tofu, tempeh, and dairy products if included in your diet. Ensure that dairy products come from ethically raised animals.

5. Balance of Satva, Rajas, and Tamas:

- The Sattvic diet seeks to balance the three gunas (qualities of nature) – Satva, Rajas, and Tamas. Satva represents purity, clarity, and harmony, while Rajas and Tamas represent restlessness and inertia, respectively.

- Choose foods that promote Satva, such as

fresh fruits, vegetables, nuts, seeds, and whole grains, while minimizing the intake of Rajasic (stimulating) and Tamasic (heavy and dull) foods.

6. Fasting and Detoxification:
   - Fasting is a common practice in many spiritual traditions. It allows the body to cleanse, purify, and rejuvenate itself while creating space for spiritual experiences.
   - Consider incorporating periodic fasting or detoxification practices under the guidance of a qualified practitioner to support spiritual growth and clarity.

7. Silence and Reflection:
   - Embrace moments of silence and reflection during your meals to deepen your connection with the divine. Avoid engaging in distracting activities or conversations while eating, allowing yourself to be fully present and attuned to your inner experiences.

8. Connection with Nature:
   - Cultivate a deep connection with nature as it fosters spiritual growth. Appreciate the natural beauty around you, spend time in serene natural settings, and honor the seasons by consuming seasonal and locally sourced foods.

9. Self-Realization and Oneness:
   - The ultimate goal of spiritual growth is self-realization and a sense of oneness with the divine. The Sattvic diet supports this journey by creating a harmonious and pure internal environment that allows for greater self-awareness and spiritual connection.

Remember, the Sattvic diet is not a guarantee of spiritual

awakening, but rather a tool that can support your spiritual journey. Along with dietary practices, embrace other spiritual disciplines such as meditation, self-inquiry, and service to others to deepen your spiritual connection and experience true awakening.

8.1 NURTURING SPIRITUALITY THROUGH SATTVIC PRACTICES

The Sattvic lifestyle encompasses more than just dietary choices. It involves a holistic approach to living that nurtures spirituality and supports the awakening of consciousness. By incorporating Sattvic practices into your daily life, you can cultivate a deeper spiritual connection, promote inner growth, and experience a sense of peace and fulfillment. Here's an extensive guide on nurturing spirituality through Sattvic practices:

1. Daily Spiritual Rituals:
    - Establish a daily routine that includes spiritual rituals such as meditation, prayer, or chanting. These practices help create a sacred space and set the tone for your day, allowing you to connect with the divine and cultivate a sense of inner peace.
    - Create a dedicated space in your home for meditation or prayer, where you can retreat and engage in these practices without distractions.

2. Mindfulness and Presence:
    - Practice mindfulness and presence in your daily activities. Whether you're eating, walking, or engaging in routine tasks,

bring your full attention to the present moment. Cultivate awareness of your thoughts, emotions, and sensations, allowing them to arise and pass without judgment.

- Engage in activities with a sense of reverence and gratitude, recognizing the divine presence in each moment.

3. Self-Reflection and Self-Inquiry:

- Set aside time for self-reflection and self-inquiry. Contemplate the deeper questions of life, explore your beliefs and values, and seek to understand the nature of your true self.

- Journaling, contemplative walks in nature, or engaging in philosophical discussions can facilitate self-reflection and the exploration of profound spiritual concepts.

4. Service and Compassion:

- Engage in acts of selfless service and cultivate compassion towards others. Volunteer, help those in need, and practice kindness and empathy in your daily interactions.

- Recognize the interconnectedness of all beings and see the divine in everyone you meet. By serving others, you not only uplift their lives but also deepen your own spiritual growth.

5. Study Sacred Texts and Wisdom:

- Engage in the study of sacred texts, spiritual teachings, and philosophical writings. Explore various spiritual traditions and seek wisdom that resonates with your soul.

- Attend lectures, workshops, or retreats led by spiritual teachers who inspire and guide you on your spiritual journey.

6. Nature Connection and Sacred Spaces:
    - Spend time in nature to connect with its inherent beauty and divinity. Take walks in serene environments, sit by a river or ocean, or immerse yourself in the tranquility of forests.

    - Create sacred spaces in your home where you can engage in spiritual practices, such as an altar adorned with meaningful symbols, candles, and sacred objects.

7. Cultivate Gratitude:
    - Practice gratitude as a way to cultivate a positive mindset and open your heart to the abundance of life. Regularly express gratitude for the blessings in your life, both big and small.

    - Keep a gratitude journal, where you write down things you're grateful for each day. This practice helps shift your focus to the positive aspects of life and deepens your spiritual connection.

8. Seek Guidance and Community:
    - Seek guidance from spiritual teachers, mentors, or elders who can offer insights and support on your spiritual journey.

    - Join spiritual communities or groups where you can engage in discussions, participate in group practices, and connect with like-minded individuals on the path of spiritual growth.

9. Inner Silence and Stillness:
    - Set aside moments of inner silence and stillness. Engage in silent meditation, contemplative walks, or simply sit in quietude, allowing your mind to settle and your true nature to emerge.

- Create space for inner listening and attuning to the wisdom that arises from deep within.

Remember, spirituality is a deeply personal and individual journey. Embrace Sattvic practices that resonate with you and adapt them to your unique path. Allow these practices to support your spiritual growth, nurture your connection with the divine, and bring a sense of peace and purpose to your life.

8.2 FASTING AND CLEANSING FOR SPIRITUAL PURIFICATION

Fasting and cleansing practices have been used for centuries as powerful tools for spiritual purification and inner transformation. By abstaining from food or engaging in detoxification rituals, individuals seek to purify their bodies, minds, and spirits, allowing for a deeper connection with the divine and a heightened state of consciousness. Here's an extensive guide on fasting and cleansing for spiritual purification:

1. Types of Fasting:
    - Water Fasting: Water fasting involves abstaining from all solid foods and consuming only water for a specific duration. It allows the body to enter a state of deep detoxification and supports spiritual purification.

    - Juice Fasting: Juice fasting involves consuming fresh fruit and vegetable juices while avoiding solid foods. It provides essential nutrients while still allowing the body to cleanse and rejuvenate.

    - Intermittent Fasting: Intermittent fasting involves restricting the eating window to a specific time frame each day, typically allowing for a period of 16-24 hours of fasting. This practice promotes cellular repair and metabolic balance.

2. Detoxification Rituals:

    - Ayurvedic Detox (Panchakarma): Panchakarma is an Ayurvedic detoxification process that involves various therapies, such as oil massages, herbal treatments, and enemas, to eliminate toxins from the body and restore balance.

    - Colon Cleansing: Colon cleansing involves removing accumulated waste and toxins from the colon through various techniques, including herbal remedies, enemas, or colon hydrotherapy. It promotes physical and energetic purification.

    - Sweating Rituals: Sweating rituals, such as saunas or sweat lodges, induce perspiration to eliminate toxins through the skin. These practices have been used in many indigenous cultures for purification and spiritual connection.

3. Intention and Mindfulness:

    - Set a clear intention for your fasting or cleansing practice. Align your intention with your spiritual goals, such as purification, clarity, or heightened awareness.

    - Practice mindfulness throughout the process. Stay present with your bodily sensations, thoughts, and emotions, observing them without attachment or judgment. Use this time to cultivate self-awareness and deepen your connection with your inner self.

4. Preparation and Gradual Transition:

- Prepare your body and mind for fasting or cleansing by gradually reducing the intake of processed foods, caffeine, and alcohol. Focus on consuming nourishing, plant-based foods to support the body's detoxification processes.

- Ease into the fasting or cleansing process by gradually reducing meal sizes or implementing intermittent fasting before engaging in longer fasts or more intense cleansing rituals.

5. Hydration and Nutrient Support:
    - During fasting or cleansing, it's essential to stay hydrated. Drink plenty of purified water, herbal teas, and fresh juices to support the body's detoxification processes and maintain proper hydration.

    - If you're engaging in longer fasts, consider supplementing with essential nutrients, such as electrolytes, vitamins, or minerals, to support the body's needs.

6. Rest and Reflection:
    - Use the fasting or cleansing period as an opportunity for rest, introspection, and self-reflection. Take time for solitude, meditation, journaling, or engaging in quiet activities that nourish your soul.

    - Allow yourself to observe any physical, emotional, or mental patterns that arise during this time. Use them as opportunities for growth, healing, and self-discovery.

7. Breaking the Fast:
    - When breaking a fast, do so gradually and mindfully. Start with small, easily digestible meals or juices and gradually reintroduce solid foods over a few days. This allows the body to

adjust and prevents digestive discomfort.

- Pay attention to how different foods impact your body and energy levels. Use this post-fast period to cultivate mindful eating habits and choose nourishing foods that support your overall well-being.

8. Spiritual Practices during Fasting or Cleansing:
    - Engage in spiritual practices that resonate with you during the fasting or cleansing period. This can include meditation, prayer, chanting, or engaging in rituals specific to your spiritual tradition.

    - Use the heightened sensitivity and clarity that often accompany fasting or cleansing to deepen your spiritual connection and engage in practices that promote inner peace, gratitude, and love.

9. Seek Professional Guidance:
    - If you're new to fasting or cleansing, or if you have any underlying health conditions, it's advisable to seek guidance from a qualified healthcare professional or a holistic practitioner experienced in fasting and cleansing practices. They can provide personalized advice and ensure your safety and well-being.

8.3 SATTVIC DIET AND CONNECTION TO HIGHER CONSCIOUSNESS

The Sattvic diet, with its emphasis on pure, fresh, and light foods, is believed to facilitate a deeper connection to higher consciousness. By aligning our dietary choices with Sattvic principles, we create an optimal environment within our bodies and minds for spiritual growth and the awakening of higher states of consciousness. Here's an extensive guide on the connection between the Sattvic diet and higher consciousness:

1. Vibrational Alignment:
    - The Sattvic diet is centered around foods that are considered to have a high vibrational frequency. These foods, such as fresh fruits and vegetables, whole grains, nuts, seeds, and legumes, are believed to carry the life force energy and nourishment needed for the body and mind to function optimally.

    - By consuming high-vibrational foods, we align ourselves with the natural rhythms of the universe and create a harmonious resonance within our being, supporting our journey towards higher consciousness.

2. Clarity and Mental Purity:

- The Sattvic diet promotes mental clarity and purity by avoiding foods that are heavy, processed, or stimulant in nature. Such foods, including meat, excessive spices, refined sugars, and caffeine, are believed to cloud the mind and hinder spiritual progress.

- By nourishing our bodies with Sattvic foods, we support the clarity of thought, enhance focus, and create a calm and balanced mental state, which is essential for accessing higher realms of consciousness.

3. Lightness and Prana:
    - Sattvic foods are known for their lightness and high pranic (life force) content. These foods are believed to nourish not only the physical body but also the subtle energy bodies, which are essential for spiritual awakening.

    - When we consume Sattvic foods, we infuse our bodies with prana, vital energy that sustains and rejuvenates us on all levels. This influx of prana nourishes the energy centers (chakras) and facilitates the flow of energy, supporting our spiritual evolution.

4. Harmonizing Body and Mind:
    - The Sattvic diet aims to create a harmonious balance between the body and mind. It recognizes the interconnectedness of physical, mental, and spiritual well-being.

    - By consuming Sattvic foods, we promote a state of equilibrium and balance within our physiological systems. This balance extends to our mental and emotional states, allowing us to experience greater peace, stability, and emotional well-being, which are conducive to higher consciousness.

5. Detoxification and Purification:

    - The Sattvic diet naturally supports the body's detoxification and purification processes. By avoiding processed, heavy, and toxic foods, we reduce the burden on our organs and facilitate the elimination of toxins from the body.

    - The purification of the physical body has a direct impact on our energy field and subtle bodies, clearing the path for the flow of higher frequencies of consciousness.

6. Sensory Discipline:

    - The Sattvic diet encourages discipline and mindfulness in our sensory experiences. It advises moderation in taste, avoiding extremes of excessively spicy, salty, or sweet foods.

    - By practicing sensory discipline, we develop greater control over our senses, reducing their influence over our thoughts and actions. This discipline supports our spiritual growth and helps us access higher states of consciousness.

7. Awareness and Mindful Eating:

    - Practicing mindfulness while consuming Sattvic foods enhances the connection between our eating experience and our spiritual journey. By eating with awareness, we engage all our senses, savor the flavors, and cultivate gratitude for the nourishment we receive.

    - Mindful eating allows us to be fully present in the moment, fostering a deeper connection with the divine within ourselves and within the food we consume.

8. Ahimsa (Non-violence) and Compassion:

- The Sattvic diet promotes the principle of ahimsa, or non-violence, by advocating a vegetarian or plant-based diet. This choice stems from the belief that consuming foods derived from the suffering or harm to sentient beings creates negative energy and hinders spiritual progress.

- By embracing a compassionate and non-violent approach to our dietary choices, we align ourselves with higher consciousness and contribute to a more harmonious and compassionate world.

9. Spiritual Practices and Integration:
   - While the Sattvic diet provides a strong foundation for spiritual growth, it is essential to complement it with other spiritual practices. Engaging in meditation, yoga, pranayama, and mindfulness practices further deepens our connection to higher consciousness and facilitates the integration of Sattvic principles into all aspects of our lives.

Embracing the Sattvic diet as part of our spiritual journey allows us to create an optimal internal environment for the awakening of higher consciousness. By choosing foods that nourish our bodies, elevate our energy, and foster mental clarity, we align ourselves with the divine and open pathways to expanded awareness, spiritual transformation, and the realization of our true nature.

CONCLUSION: EMBRACING THE SATTVIC LIFESTYLE FOR LASTING HARMONY

The Sattvic lifestyle, rooted in ancient wisdom and spiritual practices, offers a holistic approach to living in harmony with oneself, others, and the natural world. By understanding the principles and philosophy of the Sattvic diet, along with its practical applications in various aspects of life, individuals can embark on a transformative journey towards lasting harmony. Here's a comprehensive summary of the key insights gained from embracing the Sattvic lifestyle:

1. Nurturing Body, Mind, and Spirit:
    - The Sattvic lifestyle recognizes the interconnectedness of the body, mind, and spirit. By embracing a Sattvic diet and engaging in mindful eating, individuals nurture their physical well-being while supporting mental clarity and emotional balance.

    - The integration of yoga asanas, pranayama, and meditation practices further cultivates harmony between the body, mind, and spirit, leading to a more balanced and centered way of living.

2. Sattva, Rajas, and Tamas: Understanding the Three Gunas:
    - The Sattvic lifestyle acknowledges the presence of the three gunas (Sattva, Rajas, and Tamas) and seeks to cultivate Sattva, the quality of purity, balance, and harmony.
    - By consciously choosing Sattvic foods, engaging in self-reflection, and embracing mindfulness practices, individuals gradually reduce the influence of Rajas (activity) and Tamas (inertia), allowing the inherent Sattva within to shine forth.

3. Enhancing Consciousness and Self-Awareness:
    - The Sattvic lifestyle offers tools and practices to enhance consciousness and self-awareness. Through meditation, mindfulness, and self-reflection, individuals deepen their connection with their inner selves, gaining clarity, and expanding their awareness.
    - By nourishing the body with Sattvic foods and adopting a balanced daily routine, individuals create a supportive environment for personal growth, self-discovery, and the realization of their true potential.

4. Harmonizing Relationships and Creating Serenity:
    - The Sattvic lifestyle extends beyond individual well-being to encompass harmonious relationships and the creation of serene environments. By embodying qualities such as compassion, love, and non-violence (ahimsa), individuals foster harmonious interactions with others and contribute to a peaceful world.
    - Creating a Sattvic environment at home,

incorporating natural elements, and practicing self-care rituals promote a sense of tranquility, balance, and sacredness in daily life.

5. Spiritual Growth and Awakening:

    - The Sattvic lifestyle serves as a pathway for spiritual growth and awakening. By aligning with Sattvic principles, individuals cultivate a deeper connection to their spiritual essence and open themselves to higher states of consciousness.

    - Engaging in spiritual practices, such as meditation, pranayama, and the cultivation of virtues like gratitude and mindfulness, accelerates the journey towards self-realization and the recognition of the interconnectedness of all beings.

6. Integration into Modern Life:

    - The Sattvic lifestyle is adaptable and can be integrated into modern life. It encourages individuals to make conscious choices aligned with Sattvic principles in areas such as nutrition, self-care, relationships, and environmental consciousness.

    - While embracing the Sattvic lifestyle, individuals can still navigate the demands of contemporary society, finding balance, and aligning their actions with their higher values.

By embracing the Sattvic lifestyle and incorporating its principles into various aspects of life, individuals can experience a profound transformation that extends beyond physical well-being. The Sattvic lifestyle offers a path to lasting harmony, self-realization, and a deep connection to the divine essence within oneself and all of creation.

In conclusion, the Sattvic lifestyle is a profound journey of self-discovery, nourishment, and spiritual growth. It invites individuals to embody qualities of purity, balance, and harmony, fostering a deep connection to oneself, others, and the natural world. By embracing the Sattvic lifestyle, individuals can cultivate lasting harmony and embark on a transformative path towards higher consciousness, self-realization, and the realization of the interconnectedness of all beings.

GLOSSARY

1. Ahimsa - The principle of non-violence and compassion towards all living beings.

2. Chakras - Energy centers within the body associated with different aspects of physical, emotional, and spiritual well-being.

3. Gunas - The three qualities of nature: Sattva (purity), Rajas (activity), and Tamas (inertia).

4. Prana - The life force energy that sustains and vitalizes all living beings.

5. Pranayama - Breathing exercises and techniques aimed at regulating and controlling the breath and life force energy.

6. Rajas - The quality of activity, restlessness, and passion.

7. Sattva - The quality of purity, harmony, balance, and clarity.

8. Sattvic Diet - A diet consisting of pure, fresh, and light foods that promote physical, mental, and spiritual well-being.

9. Tamas - The quality of inertia, darkness, and dullness.

10. Yoga Asanas - Physical postures practiced in yoga to promote strength, flexibility, and balance.

RESOURCES FOR FURTHER EXPLORATION

For readers interested in further exploration of the Sattvic lifestyle and related topics, here are some recommended resources:

1. Books:
   - "Asana Yoga: Secrets of the Sivananda Yoga Sequence" by Jesse Danner
   - "The Yoga Sutras of Patanjali" by Swami Satchidananda
   - "The Ayurveda Bible: The Definitive Guide to Ayurvedic Healing" by Anne McIntyre
   - "The Bhagavad Gita" translated by Eknath Easwaran
   - "The Complete Book of Ayurvedic Home Remedies" by Vasant Lad
   - "The Yoga Bible" by Christina Brown

2. Websites and Online Resources:
   - The Chopra Center (www.chopra.com): Offers information on Ayurveda, meditation, and holistic well-being.
   - Yoga Journal (www.yogajournal.com): Provides articles, tutorials, and resources on yoga,

meditation, and healthy living.

- Sattvic Life (www.sattviclife.org): Offers information, recipes, and guidance on the Sattvic lifestyle and diet.
- Ayurveda.com (www.ayurveda.com): Provides comprehensive information on Ayurvedic principles, practices, and therapies.

3. Meditation and Mindfulness Apps:
   - Headspace: Offers guided meditation and mindfulness exercises for beginners and experienced practitioners.
   - Insight Timer: Provides a wide range of guided meditations, talks, and music for meditation and relaxation.
   - Calm: Offers guided meditations, breathing exercises, and sleep stories for relaxation and stress reduction.

4. Yoga and Wellness Retreats:
   - Seek out local yoga studios, wellness centers, or retreat centers that offer Sattvic lifestyle workshops, yoga retreats, and meditation retreats.
   - Look for retreats specifically focused on Ayurveda, mindfulness, or spiritual growth, where Sattvic principles are emphasized.

5. Ayurvedic Practitioners and Teachers:
   - Consider consulting with a certified Ayurvedic practitioner who can provide personalized guidance on Ayurvedic practices, including diet, herbal remedies, and lifestyle recommendations.
   - Seek out experienced yoga teachers who specialize in Sattvic practices and can guide you

in integrating Sattvic principles into your yoga and meditation practice.

Remember to approach these resources with an open mind, and always consult with healthcare professionals or experts in the field when making significant changes to your diet or lifestyle.